W9-CJZ-330

The Role of Inflammatory Mediators in the Failing Heart

Developments in Cardiovascular Medicine

208. Bernard Swynghedauw, *Molecular Cardiology for the Cardiologist, Second Edition*. 1998.   ISBN: 0-7923-8323-0
209. Geoffrey Burnstock, James G. Dobson, Jr., Bruce T. Liang, Joel Linden (eds.): *Cardiovascular Biology of Purines*. 1998. ISBN: 0-7923-8334-6
210. Brian D. Hoit, Richard A. Walsh (eds.): *Cardiovascular Physiology in the Genetically Engineered Mouse*. 1998.   ISBN: 0-7923-8356-7
211. Peter Whittaker, George S. Abela (eds.): *Direct Myocardial Revascularization: History, Methodology, Technology*. 1998. ISBN: 0-7923-8398-2
212. C.A. Nienaber, R. Fattori (eds.): *Diagnosis and Treatment of Aortic Diseases*. 1999.   ISBN: 0-7923-5517-2
213. Juan Carlos Kaski (ed.): *Chest Pain with Normal Coronary Angiograms: Pathogenesis, Diagnosis and Management*. 1999.
  ISBN: 0-7923-8421-0
214. P.A. Doevendans, R.S. Reneman and M. Van Bilsen (eds.): *Cardiovascular Specific Gene Expression*. 1999.   ISBN: 0-7923-5633-0
215. G. Pons-Lladó, F. Carreras, X. Borrás, Subirana and L.J. Jiménez-Borreguero (eds.): *Atlas of Practical Cardiac Applications of MRI*. 1999.
  ISBN: 0-7923-5636-5
216. L.W. Klein, J.E. Calvin, *Resource Utilization in Cardiac Disease*. 1999.   ISBN: 0-7923-5797-3
217. R. Gorlin, G. Dangas, P.K. Toutouzas, M.M. Konstadoulakis, *Contemporary Concepts in Cardiology, Pathophysiology and Clinical Management*.
  1999.   ISBN: 0-7923-8514-4
218. S. Gupta, J. Camm (eds.): *Chronic Infection, Chlamydia and Coronary Heart Disease*. 1999.   ISBN: 0-7923-5797-3
219. M. Rajskina, *Ventricular Fibrillation in Sudden Coronary Death*. 1999.   ISBN: 0-7923-8570-5
220. Z. Abedin, R. Conner: *Interpretation of Cardiac Arrhythmias: Self Assessment Approach*. 1999.   ISBN: 0-7923-8576-4
221. J.E. Lock, J.F. Keane, S.B. Perry: *Diagnostic and Interventional Catheterization in Congenital Heart Disease*. 2000.   ISBN: 0-7923-8597-7
222. J.S. Steinberg: *Atrial Fibrillation after Cardiac Surgery*. 2000.   ISBN: 0-7923-8655-8
223. E.E. van der Wall, A. van der Laarse, B.M. Pluim, A.V.G. Bruschke: *Left Ventricular Hypertrophy: Physiology versus Pathology*. 2000.
  ISBN: 0-7923-6038-9
224. J.F. Keaney, Jr. (ed.): *Oxidative Stress and Vascular Disease*. 2000.   ISBN: 0-7923-8678-7
228. B.E. Jaski: *Basics of Heart Failure*. 2000.   ISBN: 0-7923-7786-9
229. H.H. Osterhues, V. Hombach, A.J. Moss (eds.): *Advances in Non-Invasive Electrocardiographic Monitoring Techniques*. 2000.
  ISBN: 0-7923-6214-4
230. K. Robinson (ed.): *Homocysteine and Vascular Disease*. 2000.   ISBN: 0-7923-6248-9
231. C.I. Berul, J.A. Towbin (eds.): *Molecular Genetics of Cardiac Electrophysiology*. 2000.   ISBN: 0-7923-7829-6
232. A. Bayés de Luna, F. Furlanello, B.J. Maron and D.P. Zipes (eds.): *Arrhythmias and Sudden Death in Athletes*. 2000. ISBN: 0-7923-6337-X
233. J.-C. Tardif and M.G. Bourassa (eds.): *Antioxidants and Cardiovascular Disease*. 2000.   ISBN: 0-7923-7829-6
234. J. Candell-Riera, J. Castell-Conesa, S. Aguadé Bruiz (eds.): *Myocardium at Risk and Viable Myocardium Evaluation by SPET*. 2000.
  ISBN: 0-7923-6724-3
235. M.H. Ellestad and E. Amsterdam (eds.): *Exercise Testing: Current Concepts and Recent Advances*. 2001.   ISBN: 0-7923-7378-2

Previous volues are still available

KLUWER ACADEMIC PUBLISHERS—DORDRECHT/BOSTON/LONDON

The Role of Inflammatory Mediators in the Failing Heart

edited by

Douglas L. Mann, M.D.

Director, Winters Center for Heart Failure Research, Gordon Cain Chair and Professor of Medicine, Baylor College of Medicine, Houston, Texas

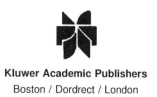

Kluwer Academic Publishers

Boston / Dordrect / London

Distributors for North, Central and South America:
Kluwer Academic Publishers
101 Philip Drive
Assinippi Park
Norwell, Massachusetts 02061 USA

Distributors for all other countries:
Kluwer Academic Publishers Group
Distribution Centre
Post Office Box 322
3300 AH Dordrecht, THE NETHERLANDS

Library of Congress Cataloging-in-Publication Data

Copyright © 2001 by Kluwer Academic Publishers

All rights reserved. No part of this publication may be reproduced, stored in a
retrieval system or transmitted in any form or by any means, mechanical,
photocopying, recording, or otherwise, without the prior written permission of the
publisher, Kluwer Academic Publishers, 101 Philip Drive, Assinippi Park, Norwell,
Massachusetts 02061

Printed on acid-free paper.

Printed in the United States of America

*The Publisher offers discounts on this book for bulk purchases. For further
information, send email to [laura.walsh@wkap.com]*

To Mark Entman and Roger Rossen, for introducing me to myocardial inflammation.

TABLE OF CONTENTS

1. The Role of Inflammatory Mediators in the Failing Heart

Introduction

" ... but when the parenchyma of the heart has been harmed by various diseases its motion is necessarily much altered; for if the parenchyma of the heart is burdened with too much fat, labours under inflammation, abscess or wound, so it cannot vibrate or contract without great trouble or difficulty, it soon gives up its motion, whence the movement of the blood also to the same degree becomes weak and languid."

Richard Lower, Tractus de Corde, 1669

Although clinicians have recognized the importance of inflammatory mediators in the pathogenesis of heart disease for well over 200 years, it has taken nearly as many years for clinicians and scientists to focus on the basic biological mechanisms by which inflammatory mediators contribute to the pathogenesis of cardiac disease states. However, over the past decade there has been increasing interest in the potential role that inflammatory mediators play in a variety of cardiac disease states, including chronic heart failure. This renewed interest has been fostered, in large measure, by the observation that many aspects of the syndrome of heart failure can be explained by the *known* biological effects of these molecules. That is, when expressed at the concentrations that are observed in heart failure, inflammatory mediators such as tumor necrosis factor, interleukin-1, interleukin-6 and nitric oxide, are sufficient to mimic some aspects of the heart failure phenotype, including (but not limited to) progressive left ventricular (LV) dysfunction, fetal gene expression, LV remodeling and cardiomyopathy. These observations have led to the suggestion that inflammatory mediators may contribute to disease progression in heart failure by virtue of the direct toxic effects that these molecules exert on the heart and the circulation.

The present issue of *Heart Failure Reviews* is an attempt to provide a structured state-of-the-art review on inflammatory mediators and the failing heart. It is my hope that this issue will serve as a useful introduction for individuals who need a comprehensive introduction to the field, as well as serve as a useful update for those colleagues who are interested in the role of inflammatory mediators and the failing heart. To this end, every effort has been made to solicit reviews from authors who have not only been in the field since its inception, but who are also capable of providing a balanced view of the relevant basic and clinical science that issues that surround this rapidly expanding and exciting field. I have also attempted to solicit relevant review articles that address the important clinical issue of the new emerging classes of therapeutic agents that can be used to modulate inflammatory mediators in the setting of heart failure. The above statements notwithstanding, the editor recognizes that it is probably not possible to cover all aspects of this rapidly changing field in a single text. Accordingly, I would like to apologize in advance to my colleagues whose outstanding contributions we were not able to recognize in the current issue of *Heart Failure Reviews*.

Douglas L. Mann, M.D.
Director,
Winters Center for Heart Failure Research,
Gordon Cain Chair and Professor of Medicine,
Baylor College of Medicine, Houston, Texas

Douglas L. Mann. THE ROLE OF INFLAMMATORY MEDIATORS IN THE FAILING HEART.
Copyright © 2001. Kluwer Academic Publishers. Boston. All rights reserved.

2. Recent Insights into the Role of Tumor Necrosis Factor in the Failing Heart

Douglas L. Mann

Winters Center for Heart Failure Research, the Cardiology Section, Department of Medicine, Veterans Administration Medical Center and Baylor College of Medicine, Houston Texas 77030

Tumor necrosis factor and the heart

Recent clinical and experimental studies have identified the importance of 'neurohormones' as biological mediators and/or modifiers of left ventricular remodeling and disease progression in the failing heart. This insight has, in turn, provided the rationale basis for antagonizing the activation of neurohormonal systems (e.g. the renin angiotensin system and the adrenergic system) in the setting of heart failure. In addition to neurohormones, it has become apparent that another portfolio of biologically active molecules, termed cytokines, are expressed along with the neurohormones in the setting of heart failure. The current interest in understanding the role or pro-inflammatory cytokines, such as tumor necrosis factor (TNF), in heart failure relates to the observation that many aspects of the syndrome of heart failure can be explained by the *known* biological effects of TNF (Table 1). Simply stated, when expressed at sufficiently high concentrations, TNF mimics some aspects of the so-called heart failure phenotype, including (but not limited to) progressive left ventricular (LV) dysfunction, pulmonary edema, LV remodeling, fetal gene expression and cardiomyopathy. Thus the elaboration of TNF, much like the elaboration of neurohormones, may represent a biological mechanism that is responsible for producing symptoms in patients with heart failure. In the present discussion, we will review several important areas that are directly relevant to the role of TNF as a mediator of disease progression in the failing heart, including a brief overview of the biology of TNF, followed by a discussion of the deleterious effects of TNF on LV remodeling effects, and finally a review of the clinical studies that link TNF production to disease progression in heart failure.

The biology of tumor necrosis factor

Tumor necrosis factor derived its name from the observation that this protein was first identified as a substance that exerted profound anti-tumor

Table 1. *The potential untoward effects of TNF in heart failure*

- Produces Left Ventricular Dysfunction
- Produces Pulmonary edema in Humans
- Produces Cardiomyopathy in Humans
- Associated with Reduced Skeletal Muscle Blood Flow in Humans
- Promotes Left Ventricular Remodeling Experimentally
- Promotes Thromboembolism Experimentally
- Produces Abnormalities in Myocardial Metabolism Experimentally
- Produces Anorexia and Cachexia Experimentally
- Produces β-receptor Uncoupling from Adenylate Cyclase Experimentally
- Abnormalities of Mitochondrial Energetics
- Activation of the Fetal Gene Program Experimentally
- Produces Cardiac Myocyte Apoptosis Experimentally

(Modified from reference [55])

effects *in vitro* and *in vivo* [1,2]. However, since this original observation, it has become clear that TNF has a variety of different biological capacities. For example, besides its cytostatic and cytotoxic effects on certain tumor cells, TNF influences growth, differentiation, and/or function of virtually every cell type investigated, including cardiac myocytes [3–5]. Although 'pro-inflammatory cytokines' such as TNF have traditionally been thought to be produced by the immune system, one of the more recent intriguing observations is that virtually all nucleated cell types within the myocardium, including cardiac myocytes themselves, are capable of synthesizing tumor necrosis factor in response to various forms of cardiac injury, including myocardial ischemia/infarction and left ventricular (LV) pressure or volume overload. Thus, from a conceptual standpoint, TNF should be envisioned as protein that is produced locally within the myocardium by 'cardiocytes' (i.e. cells that reside within the myocardium), in response to one or more different forms of environmental stress. An important corollary of this statement is that the expression of these 'stress activated'

Douglas L. Mann. THE ROLE OF INFLAMMATORY MEDIATORS IN THE FAILING HEART.
Copyright © 2001. Kluwer Academic Publishers. Boston. All rights reserved.

cytokines can occur in the complete absence of activation of immune system.

In most cell types studied TNF is initially synthesized as a nonglycosylated transmembrane protein of approximately 25 Kda. A 17 Kda fragment is proteolytically cleaved off the plasma membrane of the cell by a membrane bound enzyme termed TACE (*TNF-α convertase*) to produce the 'secreted form' of TNF, which circulates as a stable 51 Kda homotrimer. Although the literature with respect to the regulation of TNF biosynthesis in the adult heart is limited at present, at least three important themes have emerged thus far. First, neither TNF mRNA nor TNF protein appear to be constitutively expressed in the unstressed adult mammalian heart [6–8]. Second, both TNF mRNA and protein are rapidly synthesized by the heart in response to an appropriate stressful stimulus [6–8]. Third, once TNF mRNA biosynthesis is initiated, myocardial TNF mRNA levels return rapidly towards baseline following removal of the inciting stress [7]. In contrast to the findings observed in non-failing hearts, TNF mRNA and protein appear to be persistently expressed in failing human hearts. However, the mechanism for persistent TNF mRNA and protein expression in the failing heart is not known.

The effects of TNF are initiated by binding to a lower affinity ($K_d = 2$–10×10^{-10}) 55 kDa 'type 1 receptor' (also called TNFR1) and/or a higher affinity ($K_d = 2$–10×10^{-11}) 75 kDa 'type 2 receptor' (also called TNFR2). TNF induced extracellular signaling occurs as a result of TNF induced cross-linking (oligomerization) of the TNF receptors. Both TNFR1 and TNFR2 share homology in their extracellular domains, which each contain a characteristic repeated cysteine consensus motif. In contrast, the intracellular domains of TNFR1 and TNFR2 are different, suggesting that each receptor has distinct modes of signaling and cellular function. Previous studies have identified the presence of both types of TNF receptors in non-failing [9] and failing human myocardium [10]; in addition, the presence of TNFR1 has been identified recently in rat cardiac myocytes [11]. Although, the exact functional significance of TNFR1 and TNFR2 in the heart is not known at present, as shown in Table 2 the majority of the deleterious effects of TNF are coupled to activation of TNFR1, whereas activation of TNFR2 appears to exert protective effects in the heart. Activation of TNFR1 is responsible for mediating negative inotropic effects [9] through activation of the neutral sphingomyelinase pathway [12], cardiac myocyte apoptosis, and increased HSP 72 expression [13]. In contrast, activation of the type 2 TNF receptor appears to protect the myocyte against hypoxic stress and ischemic injury [14], but has no effect on cell motion.

Tumor necrosis factor and left ventricular remodeling

For the purpose of the present review we will define LV remodeling as a change in LV chamber and volume that is not related to pre-load mediated increase in sarcomere length [15,16]. While the complex changes that occur in the heart during left ventricular remodeling have commonly been described in mechanical and/or anatomic terms, left ventricular remodeling involves important alterations in the biology of the cardiac myocyte, changes in volume of myocyte and non-myocyte components of the myocardium, as well as alterations in the chamber geometry and architecture of the heart. As shown in Table 3, TNF stimulation evokes a number of important effects on cardiac myocyte biology, cardiac matrix biology, as well as alterations in LV chamber geometry. Accordingly, we will attempt to discuss those TNF induced changes that occur in the cardiac myocyte, the myocardium and the LV chamber that are directly relevant to the process of LV remodeling.

TNF induced changes in cardiac myocytes
TNF stimulation of isolated cardiac myocytes provokes at least three changes in cardiac

Table 2. *Biological effects of TNF receptors in the adult mammalian heart*

TNF Receptor Subtype	Response in Cardiac Myocytes
TNFR1 (p55)	• Negative inotropic effects [9] • Activation of HSP 72 [56] • Cytoprotection [57] • Apoptosis of cardiac myocytes [13]
TNFR2 (p75)	• Cytoprotection [14]

Table 3. *Effects of TNF on left ventricular remodeling*

- Alterations in the Biology of the Myocyte
  - Myocyte Hypertrophy
  - Contractile Abnormalities
  - Fetal Gene Expression
- Alteration in the Extracellular Matrix
  - Degradation of the Matrix
  - Replacement Fibrosis
- Progressive Myocyte Loss
  - Necrosis
  - Apoptosis

myocytes that are relevant to the process of LV remodeling; namely myocyte hypertrophy [3], progressive myocyte cell death through apoptosis [13], contractile defects, as well as alterations in fetal gene expression [17,18]. Although the effects of TNF on cardiac myocyte hypertrophy are relatively modest, the extant literature suggests that stimulation with TNF increases sarcomeric protein synthesis in cultured adult cardiac myocytes [3]. Relevant to this discussion is the observation that TNF is sufficient to provoke cardiac myocyte hypertrophy in experimental models wherein TNF was infused at pathophysiologically relevant concentrations [19], as well as in transgenic mice that harbor cardiac restricted overexpression of TNF [17]. TNF has also been shown to trigger apoptosis in isolated cardiac myocytes through activation of the neutral sphingomyelinase pathway. Finally, TNF has been shown to provoke negative inotropic effects in isolated cardiac myocytes through a variety of different mechanisms (reviewed in reference [20]). For example, the extant literature suggests that TNF provokes *immediate* negative inotropic effects in myocytes that are mediated, at least in part, by the neutral sphingomyelinase pathway, as well as *delayed* negative inotropic effects that are mediated by nitric oxide. In addition, it has been shown that sustained expression of TNF can lead to down regulation of SERCA2A, which is responsible for calcium homeostasis in the cardiac myocyte [18]. Thus, the mechanism for TNF induced contractile dysfunction is likely to be far more complex than was originally thought.

In addition to the changes in the biology of the myocyte discussed above, TNF may also alter cardiac myocyte metabolism. Although systematic studies of the effects of TNF on cardiac myocyte metabolism have not been performed, it is important to recognize that TNF increases lipoprotein lipase activity in the hearts of mice, rats and guinea pigs *in vivo* [21]. In addition, TNF is known to interfere with insulin metabolism in a variety of mammalian cells [22–24]. Although speculative, it is possible that altered expression of lipoprotein lipase or insulin metabolism in the failing heart may lead to increases in triglyceride-derived free fatty acid availability and utilization. An increase in the metabolism of free-fatty acids might be expected to produce deleterious effects in the failing heart by increasing myocardial oxygen demand. In support of this statement is a recent experimental study in dogs, wherein an infusion of free fatty acids in an ischemic dog heart produced a significant worsening of LV function with a resultant increase in LV dilatation [25]. Thus, it is conceivable that TNF may adversely affect the biology of the cardiac myocyte through alterations in the metabolism of the myocyte.

TNF induced changes in the extracellular matrix

Several lines of evidence suggest that TNF may promote left ventricular remodeling through alterations in the extracellular matrix component of the myocardium. First, when human volunteers were administered endotoxin (a potent stimulus for TNF production) intravenously, there was ≈ 20% increase in left ventricular end-diastolic volume within five hours [26]. Moreover, the changes in LV volume in the endotoxin treated subjects did not appear to be due either to changes in pre-load or afterload. Second, a recent experimental study [19] shows that there was a time dependent change in LV dimension (Figure 1) that was accompanied by progressive degradation of the extracellular matrix (Figure 2) in rats that were infused with concentrations of TNF that are observed in patients with heart failure. Moreover, similar findings have been reported following a single infusion of TNF in dogs [27]. Finally, a recent study by Kubota et al. showed that a transgenic mouse line that overexpressed TNF in the cardiac compartment developed progressive LV dilation over a 24 week period of observation [17]. Similar findings have also been reported by Bryant et al. [28], who targeted TNF overexpression in the heart and observed identical findings with respect to LV dysfunction and LV dilation. As shown by the Magnetic Resonance images in Figure 3, transgenic mice overexpressing TNF in the cardiac compartment develop progressive LV dilation. Although these studies did not elucidate the changes for the TNF induced increase in LV dimension, it is interesting to note that both IL-1β and TNF are capable of activating a family of collagenolytic enzymes referred to as matrix metalloproteinases [29–31], that are responsible for degrading the extracellular matrix. Relevant to this discussion is the observation by Weber and colleagues that type 1 collagen weave is disrupted in myocardial samples taken from patients with dilated cardiomyopathy [32]. Dissolution of the type 1 collagen weave that surrounds the individual cardiac myocytes and links the myocytes together has been suggested to result in a loss of force development in the heart [33,34], as well as allow for rearrangement ('slippage') of bundles or groups of cardiac myocytes [34]. Thus, excessive activation of proinflammatory cytokines may contribute to LV remodeling through a variety of different mechanisms that involve both the myocyte and non-myocyte components of the heart.

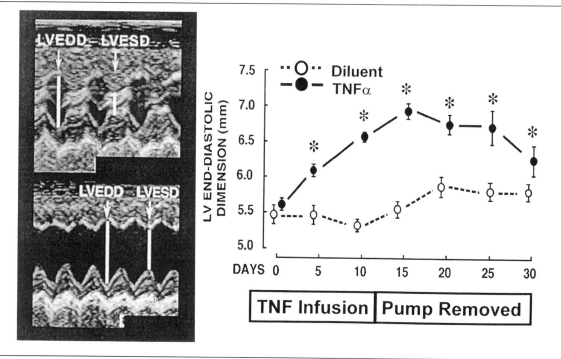

Fig. 1. *Effect of a continuous TNF infusion in vivo, on LV structure in rats. LV dimensions were determined in rats that underwent implantation of an intraperitoneal osmotic infusion pump that contained wither diluent or TNF. The amount of TNF in the osmotic infusion pumps was titrated to achieve systemic levels that are observed in patients with heart failure (≈ 80–100 U/ml). After 15 days the osmotic infusion pumps were removed and the animals were allowed to recover. LV dimensions were assessed serially at baseline and every 5 days for a total of 30 days, using echocardiography to measure LV internaol dimensions. As shown, there was progressive LV dilation in the animals that received a continuous infusion of TNF, whereas there was no significant change in LV dimension in the animals that received diluent alone. Further, there was very little regression in LV dilation after the osmotic pumps were removed, suggesting that the TNF infusion had led to alteration in the structural integrity of the heart. (Reproduced with permission from Bozkurt et al. [19] the American Heart Association).*

TNF induced changes in the left ventricular geometry

Previous experimental studies have consistently shown that simulation with TNF produces an increase in LV cavity dimension and LV wall thinning [17,19,27,28]. While the mechanisms that are responsible for these potentially deleterious changes are likely to be very complex, they are likely to involve TNF-induced changes in the biology of the myocyte (hypertrophy and apoptosis), as well as TNF induced changes in the extracellular matrix (degradation of fibrillar collagen).

Elaboration and functional significance of TNF in human heart failure

In an effort to define a biochemical mechanism for cardiac cachexia, Levine et al. made the sentinel observation that patients with advanced heart failure (NYHA class III–IV) expressed elevated levels of biologically active TNF in their peripheral circulation [35]. The notion that TNF might play a role in cardiac cachexia was also suggested in a subsequent paper by

McMurray and colleagues [36], who reported that elevated levels of TNF were found in nine of 16 patients with cachexia, whereas only one of 10 patients without cardiac cachexia had an elevated level of TNF. Additional reports by Anker and colleagues have confirmed the relationship between TNF and cardiac cachexia [37]. Taken together, these studies suggest that overexpression of TNF may contribute to systemic wasting in advanced heart failure. However, it has also become abundantly clear that the elaboration of TNF is also observed in direct relation to NYHA functional class in patients with heart failure, and not strictly in patients with cachexia [38–40]. Thus, as will be discussed below, it is likely that TNF may play a much broader role heart failure than was originally posited.

The functional role of TNF in modulating myocardial structure and function was originally suggested by studies by Torre-Amione et al. who observed that TNF mRNA and protein were expressed in the myocardium of patients with both ischemic and dilated cardiomyopathy [10]. Since this observation, two other laboratories

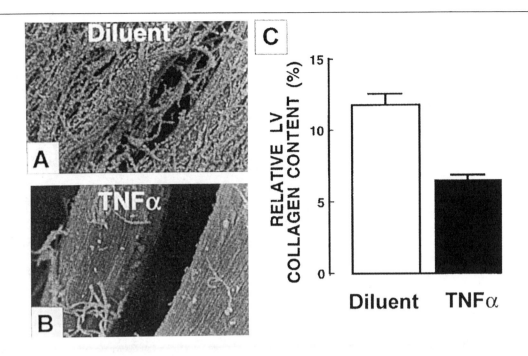

Fig. 2. *Effect of TNF infusion on collagen content of the heart. LV collagen content was examined in rats that underwent implantation of an intraperitoneal osmotic infusion pumps that contained wither diluent or TNF. The amount of TNF in the osmotic infusion pumps was titrated to achieve systemic levels that are observed in patients with heart failure (≈ 80–$100\,U/ml$). After 15 days the osmotic infusion pumps were removed and the animals were allowed to recover. LV dimensions collagen content was assessed at baseline and at 15 days using the picrosirius red technique. Panel A shows a scanning electron microscopic picture of myocardial tissue from an animal that received dluent for 15 days; panel B shows a scanning electron microscopic picture of myocardial tissue from an animal that received TNF for 15 days. As shown, there was a striking loss of the collagen weave surrounding the myocytes in the animals that had received an infusion of TNF. Panel C depicts the results of group data and shows thata TNF infusion was associated with $\approx 50\%$ decrease in the collagen content of the heart, thus suggesting that disruptionof the collagen content of the heart may have contributed to the observed LV dilation in the TNF treated hearts. (Modified from Bozkurt et al. [19] the American Heart Association).*

have confirmed this result [41,42]. Although the functional significance of TNF in the failing heart is not known at present, the observation that TNF can mimic many aspects of the heart failure phenotype (Table 1, 3), has raised the interesting possibility that when TNF is overexpressed in the myocardium that it might contribute to the process LV remodeling. This statement is supported by the recent preliminary report that administration of a soluble TNF antagonist was sufficient to lead to increased pump performance as well as a decrease in LV end-diastolic dimension in patients with NYHA class III/IV heart failure [43].

The functional role of TNF in modulating endothelial function is suggested by studies in a report by Katz et al. who showed that the elevated levels of TNF in heart failure patients (class II–III) correlated with the forearm blood flow responses to acetylcholine and nitroglycerin. These authors postulated that increased levels of TNF in heart failure patients might serve to partially compensate for the previously reported

decrease in vasodilatory response to activation of cNOS that has been reported in this syndrome [44]. In a separate report by Agnoletti et al. [45], it was subsequently shown that serum from patients with heart failure patients was sufficient to down-regulate endothelial constitutive nitric oxide synthase (eNOS) and induce apoptosis in cultured human endothelial cells. Relevant to the present discussion was the observation that an anti-human TNF antibody partially counteracted these deleterious effects, suggesting that TNF was a circulating factor that contributed to the endothelial dysfunction observed in this study. This concept is further supported by studies by Anker and colleagues [46], who showed that circulating levels of TNF correlated inversely with peak blood flow in heart failure patients, independently of age, ejection fraction, peak oxygen consumption, and NYHA association class, thus suggesting that TNF induced endothelial dysfunction might be related to peripheral skeletal muscle weakness/fatigue in patients with heart failure.

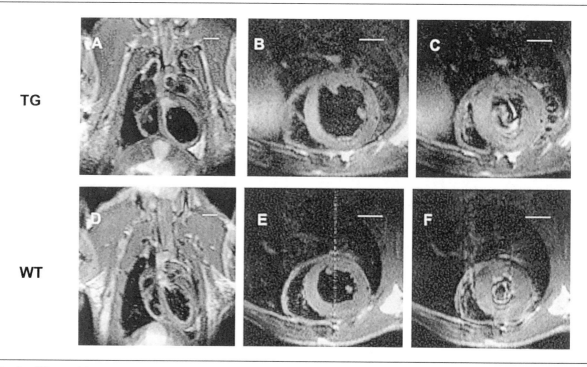

Fig. 3. *LV remodeling in a transgenic mouse model of TNF overexpression. TNF overexpression was targetted to the cardiac compartment of transgenic mice. Magnetic resonance images of the heart were obtained from 24 week old transgenic mice (panel A, B, and C) and an age-matched control mouse (panel D, E, F). As shown, there was signficant LV dilation in the animal harbouring the TNF transgene in the cardiac compartment. (Reproduced with permission from Kobuta et al. [17], the American Heart Association).*

Do elevated proinflammatory cytokine levels have prognostic importance?

The question as to whether proinflammatory cytokine levels correlate with patient prognosis has been addressed in several studies. To determine whether there was a relationship between patient survival and TNF levels, a Kaplan-Meier analysis was performed for SOLVD patients in whom cytokine levels had been determined [38]. At the end of the 48 month follow-up period for the SOLVD patients, 14 patients (22.2%) had died and 49 (77.8%) patients with NYHA class I–III remained alive. As shown in Figure 4, when patients with TNF levels > 6.6 pg/ml (90th percentile) were examined, there was a significant increase in overall patient mortality when compared to patients with TNF levels < 6.5 pg/ml. However, these data must be regarded as provisional, since the overall patient cohort was relatively small and relatively select. Nonetheless, these data suggest that vasodepressor cytokines such as TNF may have prognostic significance in heart failure. Ferrari and colleagues [45] observed that levels of TNF and sTNFR2 were significantly higher in hospitalized patients with the worst clinical outcomes, and that elevated levels of sTNFR2 were the single

most important variable predicting patient death in a stepwise discriminant analysis. Thus, there is increasing evidence that elevated levels of TNF may correlate with patient prognosis.

What is the Site and Source of tumor necrosis factor in heart failure?

Following the original descriptions of elevated cytokine levels in cachectic patients with heart failure, one of the more intriguing challenges that arose was to identify the mechanism(s) that was responsible for the production of inflammatory mediators in heart failure. As shown in Table 4 there are at least five hypotheses with respect to the source of production for proinflammatory cytokines in heart failure. The original suggestion with regard to the mechanism for cytokine overproduction was that these molecules were produced secondary to the 'immune activation' that occurred in response to tissue injury [47]. This concept was subsequently challenged by the observation from several laboratories that TNF and nitric oxide synthase were expressed by in the failing human heart in the absence of a demonstrable inflammatory infiltrate, suggesting that the heart was a potential source of produc-

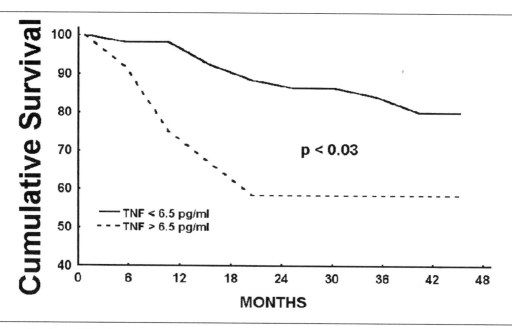

Fig. 4. *Prognostic values of TNF levels. A Kaplan–Meier analysis was performed for SOLVD pateints with TNF levels less than or greater than 6.5 pg/ml (90th percentile). As shown, there was a significant increase in overall patient mortality for pateints with TNF levels > 6.5 pg/ml when compared to pateints with TNF levels < 6.5 pg/ml. (Reproduced with permission from reference Seta et al. [58] the Journal of Cardiac Failure).*

tion of inflammatory mediators [9]. A third hypothesis suggests that the elaboration of cytokines is the result of underperfusion of systemic tissues [48,49]. While this may be true for IL-6 production, there is no evidence that the increase in TNF production is the result of increased peripheral arteriovenous production [49]. More recently it has been suggested that increased bowel wall edema in patients with heart failure leads to translocation of bacterial endotoxin from the gut, with resultant activation of the immune system [50]. While the 'endotoxin hypothesis' remains as an attractive explanation for the elaboration of cytokines in edematous patients with advanced heart failure, this mechanism does not account for the elaboration of cytokines in patients with milder forms of heart failure, who are edema free [38,51]. Finally, it has been shown in cell culture models that increased levels of cAMP will serve to stabilize the mRNA for several inflammatory mediators, most notably nitric oxide synthase [52]. This, in turn, has given rise to the suggestion that the adrenergic

nervous system may serve to augment cytokine production in the setting of heart failure. Experimental studies have shown that administration of β-blockers in the post-infarct setting will attenuate myocardial cytokine production, while administration of isoproterenol provokes myocardial cytokine production [53,54]. However, given that agents that increase cAMP are known to block cytokine production, it is unclear at the time of this writing whether this explanation will prove to be an important mechanism for the increased elaboration in the setting of heart failure. Given that no single mechanism described above is sufficient to explain the production of cytokines in the setting of heart failure, it is unlikely that we will ever identify a single site or source of cytokine production in the disease state that is as complex as heart failure. Indeed, it is becoming increasingly likely that there will be multiple sites and sources of cytokine production as heart failure advances, analogous to the situation with activation of the renin angiotensin system and the adrenergic system, both of which are activated in an extremely complex manner as heart failure progresses.

Table 4. *Potential sites and sources for cytokine elaboration in heart failure*

- Immune activation
- Myocardial biosynthesis
- Hypoperfusion of metabolic tissue
- Endotoxin absorption from the gut
- Adrenergic stimulation

Conclusion

In the present review we have focused on recent clinical and experimental evidence which suggests that TNF may play a role in disease progression in heart failure, by virtue of the direct toxic effects that this molecule exerts in the heart and the peripheral circulation. The extant literature suggests that pathophysiologically relevant concentrations of TNF mimic many aspects of the heart failure phenotype in experimental animals, including LV dysfunction, LV dilation, activation of fetal gene expression, cardiac myocyte hypertrophy and cardiac myocyte apoptosis (Table 1, 3). The extant clinical literature suggests that TNF may play a role in the process of LV remodeling, as well as the endothelial dysfunction that is observed in heart failure. Thus, analogous to the proposed role for neurohormones, TNF would appear to represent another distinct class of biologically active molecules that can contribute to heart failure progression. As will be discussed later in this review, there is increasing evidence which suggest that circulating levels of cytokines can be antagonized effectively through a variety of different 'targeted' strategies. While it is perhaps premature to speculate whether modulating cytokine levels will translate into clinical improvements in morbidity and mortality for patients with heart failure, there is now a growing body of evidence which suggests that modulating cytokine levels may represent a new therapeutic paradigm for treating patients with heart failure.

Acknowledgments

The author would like to thank Mary Helen Soliz for secretarial assistance, as well as Dr. Andrew I. Schafer for his past and present guidance and support. The research reviewed herein was supported, in part, by research funds from the Department of Veterans Affairs and the N.I.H. (P50 HL-O6H and RO1 HL58081-01, RO1 HL61543-01, HL-42250-10/10).

References

1. Carswell EA, Old LJ, Kassel RL, et al. An endotoxin-induced serum factor that causes necrosis of tumors. *Proc Natl Acad Sci USA* 1975;72:3666–3670.
2. Old LJ. Tumor necrosis factor (TNF). *Science* 1985;230:630–632.
3. Yokoyama T, Nakano M, Bednarczyk JL, et al. Tumor necrosis factor-α provokes a hypertrophic growth response in adult cardiac myocytes. *Circulation* 1997;95:1247–1252.
4. Yokoyama T, Vaca L, Rossen RD, et al. Cellular basis for the negative inotropic effects of tumor necrosis factor-alpha in the adult mammalian heart. *J Clin Invest* 1993;92:2303–2312.
5. Gulick TS, Chung MK, Pieper SJ, et al. Interleukin 1 and tumor necrosis factor inhibit cardiac myocyte β-adrenergic responsiveness. *Proc Natl Acad Sci USA* 1989;86:6753–6757.
6. Giroir BP, Johnson JH, Brown T, et al. The tissue distribution of tumor necrosis factor biosynthesis during endotoxemia. *J Clin Invest* 1992;90:693–698.
7. Kapadia S, Lee JR, Torre-Amione G, et al. Tumor necrosis factor gene and protein expression in adult feline myocardium after endotoxin administration. *J Clin Invest* 1995;96:1042–1052.
8. Kapadia S, Oral H, Lee J, et al. Hemodynamic regulation of tumor necrosis factor-α gene and protein expression in adult feline myocardium. *Circ Res* 1997;81:187–195.
9. Torre-Amione G, Kapadia S, Lee J, et al. Expression and functional significance of tumor necrosis factor receptors in human myocardium. *Circulation* 1995;92:1487–1493.
10. Torre-Amione G, Kapadia S, Lee J, et al. Tumor necrosis factor-α and tumor necrosis factor receptors in the failing human heart. *Circulation* 1996;93:704–711.
11. Krown KA, Yasui K, Brooker MJ, et al. TNFα receptor expression in rat cardiac myocytes: TNFα inhibition of L-type Ca^{2+} current and Ca^{2+} transients. *FEBS Lett* 1995;376:24–30.
12. Oral H, Dorn GW, II, Mann DL. Sphingosine mediates the immediate negative inotropic effects of tumor necrosis factor-α in the adult mammalian cardiac myocyte. *J Biol Chem* 1997;272:4836–4842.
13. Krown KA, Page MT, Nguyen C, et al. Tumor necrosis factor alpha-induced apoptosis in cardiac myocytes: involvement of the sphingolipid signaling cascade in cardiac cell death. *J Clin Invest* 1996;98:2854–2865.
14. Nakano M, Knowlton AA, Dibbs Z, et al. Tumor necrosis factor-α confers resistance to injury induced by hypoxic injury in the adult mammalian cardiac myocyte. *Circulation* 1998;97:1392–1400.
15. Linzbach AJ. Heart Failure from the Point of View of Quantitative Anatomy. *Am J Cardiol* 1960;69:370–382.
16. Cohn JN. Structural basis for heart failure: Ventricular remodeling and its pharmacological inhibition. *Circulation* 1995;91:2504–2507.
17. Kubota T, McTiernan CF, Frye CS, et al. Dilated cardiomyopathy in transgenic mice with cardiac specific overexpression of tumor necrosis factor-alpha. *Circ Res* 1997;81:627–635.
18. Kubota T, Bounoutas GS, Miyagishima M, et al. Soluble tumor necrosis factor receptor abrogates myocardial inflammation but not hypertrophy in cytokine-induced cardiomyopathy. *Circulation* 2000; 101(21):2518–2525.
19. Bozkurt B, Kribbs S, Clubb Jr FJ, et al. Patho physiologically relevant concentrations of tumor necrosis factor-α promote progressive left ventricular dysfunction and remodeling in rats. *Circulation* 1998; 97:1382–1391.
20. Mann DL. Cytokines as mediators of disease progression in the failing heart. In: Hosenpud JD, Greenberg BH, eds. *Congestive Heart Failure*. Philadelphia: Lippincott Williams & Wilkins, 1999:213–232.
21. Semp H, Peterson J, Tavernier J, et al. Multiple effects of tumor necrosis factor on lipoprotein lipase *in vivo*. *J Biol Chem* 1987;262:8390–8395.
22. Begum N, Ragolia L. Effect of tumor necrosis factor-α on insulin action in cultured rat skeletal muscle cells. *Endocrinology* 1996;137:2441–2446.
23. Peraldi P, Hotamisligil GS, Buurman WA, et al. Tumor necrosis factor (TNF)-alpha inhibits insulin signaling through stimulation of the p55 TNF receptor and

activation of sphingomyelinase. *J Biol Chem* 1996; 271:13018–13022.

24. Lang CH, Dobrescu C, Bagby GJ. Tumor necrosis factor impairs insulin action on peripheral glucose disposal and hepatic glucose output. *Endocrinology* 1992;130:43–52.
25. Kjekshus J, Mjos O. Effects of free fatty acids on myocardial function and metabolism in the ischemic dog heart. *J Clin Invest* 1994;51:1767–1776.
26. Suffredini AF, Fromm RE, Parker MM, et al. The cardiovascular response of normal humans to the administration of endotoxin. *N Engl J Med* 1989; 321:280–287.
27. Pagani FD, Basker LS, Hsi C, et al. Left ventricular systolic and diastolic dysfunction after infusion of tumor necrosis factor-α in conscious dogs. *J Clin Invest* 1992;90:389–398.
28. Bryant D, Becker L, Richardson J, et al. Cardiac Failure in transgenic mice with myocardial expression of tumor necrosis factor-α (TNF). *Circulation* 1998; 97:1375–1381.
29. Sciavolino PJ, Lee TH, Vilcek J. Interferon-β induces metalloproteinase mRNA expression in human fibroblasts. *J Biol Chem* 1994;269:21627–21634.
30. Van der Zee E, Everts V, Beertsen W. Cytokines modulate routes of collagen breakdown: review with special emphasis of collagen degradation in the periodontium and the burst hypothesis of periodontal disease progression. *J Clin Periodontol* 1997; 24:297–305.
31. Rawdanowicz TJ, Hampton AL, Nagase H, et al. Matrix metalloproteinase production by cultured human endometrial stromal cells: identification of interstitial collagenase, gelatinase-A, genatinase-B, and stromelysin-1 and their differential regulation by interleukin-1α and their differential regulation by interleukin-1α and tumor necrosis factor-α. *J Clin Endocrinol Metab* 1994;79:530–536.
32. Weber KT, Pick R, Janicki JS, et al. Inadequate collagen tethers in dilated cardiopathy. *Am Heart J* 1998;116:1641–1646.
33. Factor SM, Robinson TF. Comparative connective tissue structure: function relationships in biological pumps. *Lab Invest* 1988;58:150–156.
34. Weber KT. Cardiac Interstitium in Health and Disease: The Fibrillar Collagen Networks. *J Am Coll Cardiol* 1989;13(7):1637–1652.
35. Levine B, Kalman J, Mayer L, et al. Elevated circulating levels of tumor necrosis factor in severe chronic heart failure. *N Engl J Med* 1990;223:236–241.
36. McMurray J, Abdullah I, Dargie HJ, et al. Increased concentrations of tumor necrosis factor in 'cachetic' patients with severe chronic heart failure. *Br Heart J* 1991;66:356–358.
37. Anker SD, Ponikowski P, Varney S, et al. Wasting as independent risk factor for mortality in chronic heart failure. *Lancet* 1997;349:1050–1053.
38. Torre-Amione G, Kapadia S, Benedict CR, et al. Proinflammatory cytokine levels in patients with depressed left ventricular ejection fraction: a report from the studies of left ventricular dysfunction (SOLVD). *J Am Coll Cardiol* 1996;27:1201–1206.
39. Testa M, Yeh M, Lee P, et al. Circulating levels of cytokines and their endogenous modulators in patients with mild to severe congestive heart failure due to coronary artery disease or hypertension. *J Am Coll Cardiol* 1996;28:964–971.
40. Bachetti T, Comini L, Agnoletti L, et al. Attivazione e ruolo del fattore di necrosi tumorale alfa nello scompenso cardiaco congestizio. *Cardiologia* 1996;41:343–347.
41. Doyama K, Fujiwara H, Fukumoto M, et al. Tumour necrosis factor is expressed in cardiac tissues of patients with heart failure. *Int J Cardiol* 1996; 54(3):217–225.
42. Habib FM, Springall DR, Davies GJ, et al. Tumour necrosis factor and inducible nitric oxide synthase in dilated cardiomyopathy. *Lancet* 1996;347:1151–1155.
43. Bozkurt B, Torre-Amione G, Deswal A, Soran OZ, Whitmore J, Warren M, Mann DL. Regression of left ventricular remodeling in chronic heart failure after treatment with enbrel (Etanercept, p75 TNF receptor Fc fusion protein). *Circulation* 100:I, 105. 1999. Ref Type: Generic.
44. Katz SD, Rao R, Berman JW, et al. Pathophysiological correlates of increased serum tumor necrosis factor in patients with congestive heart failure: relation to nitric oxide-dependent vasodilation in the forearm circulation. *Circulation* 1994;90:12–16.
45. Ferrari R, Bachetti T, Confortini R, et al. Tumor necrosis factor soluble receptors in patients with various degrees of congestive failure. *Circulation* 1995;92:1479–1486.
46. Anker SD, Volterrnani M, Egerer KR, et al. TNF-α as predictor of peak leg blood flow in chronic heart failure. *Q J Med* 1998;91:199–203.
47. Matsumori A, Yamada T, Suzuki H, et al. Increased circulating cytokines in patients with myocarditis and cardiomyopathy. *Br Heart J* 1994;72;561–566.
48. Sindhwani R, Yuen J, Hirsch H, Tegguy A, Galvao M, Levato P, LeJemtel TH. Reversal of low flow state attenuates immune activation in severe decompensated congestive heart failure. *Circulation* 1993; 88:I-255.
49. Tsutamoto T, Hisanaga T, Wada A, et al. Interleukin-6 spillover in the peripheral circulation increases with the severity of heart failure, and the high plasma level of interleukin-6 is an important prognostic predictor in patients with congestive heart failure. *J Am Coll Cardiol* 1998;31:391–398.
50. Niebauer J, Volk H-D, Kemp M, et al. Endotoxin and immune activation in chronic heart failure: a prospective cohort study. *Lancet* 99 A.D.;353:1838–1842.
51. Dibbs Z, Thornby J, White BG, et al. Natural Variability of Circulating Levels of Cytokines and Cytokine Receptors in Patients with Heart Failure: Implications for Clinical Trials. *J Am Coll Cardiol* 1999; 33:1935–1942.
52. Oddis CV, Simmons RL, Hattler BG, et al. cAMP enhances inducible nitric oxide synthase mRNA stability in cardiac myocytes. *Am J Physiol* 1995;269:H2044–H2050.
53. Murray DR, Prabhu SD, Chandrasekar B. Chronic beta-adrenergic stimulation induces myocardial proinflammatory cytokine expression. *Circulation* 2000;101(20):2338–2341.

54. Prabhu SD, Chandrasekar B, Murray DR, et al. Beta-adrenergic blockade in developing heart failure: effects on myocardial inflammatory cytokines, nitric oxide, and remodeling. *Circulation* 2000; 101(17):2103–2109.

55. Kapadia S, Dibbs Z, Kurrelmeyer K, et al. The role of cytokines in the failing human heart. In: Crawford M, ed. *Cardiology Clinics.* Philadelphia: W.B. Saunders, 1998:645–656.

56. Nakano M, Knowlton AA, Yokoyama T, et al. Tumor necrosis factor-α induced expression of heat shock protein 72 in adult feline cardiac myocytes. *Am J Physiol* 1996;270:H1231–H1239.

57. Kurrelmeyer K, Michael L, Baumgarte G, et al. Endogenous myocardial tumor necrosis factor protects the adult cardiac myocyte against ischemic-induced apoptosis in a murine model of acute myocardial infarction. *Proc Natl Acad Sci USA* 2000;290:5456–5461.

58. Seta Y, Shan K, Bozkurt B, et al. Basic mechanisms in heart failure: the cytokine hypothesis. *J Cardiac Failure* 1996;2:243–249.

3. The Role of Interleukin-1 in the Failing Heart

Carlin S. Long, MD

Cardiology Section, Denver Health Medical Center and the
University of Colorado, Denver, CO 80204

Introduction

Although the last ten years have seen dramatic improvements in the therapeutic approach to CHF, the expanding number of those afflicted with this disease and its persistent poor prognosis make it clear that additional novel approaches are necessary. In this regard, there has recently been an increasing appreciation of an important inflammatory component in both the development and progression of the failing heart. Specifically, increased levels of several pro-inflammatory cytokines have been found to be elevated in patients with advanced stage disease and these levels appear to correlate with a worse prognosis. This has lead to the description of the 'cytokine hypothesis' of myocardial dysfunction in which myocardial injury is associated with the elaboration of pro-inflammatory molecules by both immune effector cells, as well as cells intrinsic to the heart itself (Fig. 1). These cytokines then act in both a paracrine (cardiac myocyte) and autocrine (cardiac fibroblast) manner to augment the changes in myocardial phenotype and function characteristic of the failing heart. As an example of potential autocrine action, many cytokines have direct effects on extracellular matrix homeostasis. Accordingly, a role in the myocardial remodeling that occurs following injury/infarction has been suggested [1–3]. As such, if the local expression of cytokines can be targeted therapeutically, the myocardial response to injury at the level of both acute dysfunction as well as the subsequent remodeling could be modified.

In this chapter and the others in this volume, the possibility that specific molecules in the pro-inflammatory cascade play a substantive role in both the development and progression of myocardial disease states is explored. Further, it is the firm belief of the Authors in this volume that the cytokines investigated, as well as their respective signaling pathways, are viable targets for treating heart failure, an hypothesis that is supported by the recent work using a cytokine-targeted strategy.

Although there are many 'reactive' cytokines, it is generally felt that the induction of the pro-inflammatory cascade follows the production of three main cytokines, namely interleukin-1

(IL-1), tumor necrosis factor (TNF), and interleukin-6 (IL-6). In view of the effects of IL-1 on myocyte growth and gene expression observed by both our lab and others [4–10], our research group has chosen to focus primarily on the role of this cytokine in the failing heart. This being said, it is a given that there is no *one* cytokine that leads to the development and/or progression of the heart failure syndrome. Rather, it is likely that it is the composite effects of the pro-inflammatory cascade and their downstream effectors that *together* produce alterations in myocardial function.

Herein we survey the data supporting a role for IL-1 in the failing heart and discuss potential transcriptional mechanisms of the IL-1 effect using an *in vitro* model system. The organization of this review starts with the observational data in human and experimental myocardial dysfunction supporting a substantive role for IL-1. These observations from the foundation for the subsequent description of the more mechanistic investigations into IL-1 action on the heart.

IL-1 in the human heart

IL-1 has been implicated in the pathogenesis of several different types of myocardial dysfunction in man. Many of these investigations have relied upon levels of IL-1 in the circulation of patients with these syndromes. However, additional *in vitro* work has been performed suggesting that a cause and effect relationship may, in fact, exist. In one of the first reports on IL-1 expression in the heart, Han et al. found that hearts of patients with idiopathic dilated cardiomyopathy contained an increase in IL-1β expression [11]. Similar results were reported by Francis et al. [12] and IL-1 has also been found in hearts of patients with viral myocarditis [13,14]. Increased circulating levels of IL-1 have been found in patients with congestive heart failure, acute rheumatic fever, stable/unstable coronary syndromes, post-cardiopulmonary bypass, following transplantation/transplant rejection and, of course, sepsis [15–19].

In addition, several *in vitro* investigations using material isolated from human heart has confirmed a detrimental effect for IL-1 on contractile function. In one such study, Cain

Douglas L. Mann. *THE ROLE OF INFLAMMATORY MEDIATORS IN THE FAILING HEART.*
Copyright © 2001. Kluwer Academic Publishers. Boston. All rights reserved.

The Cytokine Hypothesis of Myocardial Dysfunction

Myocardial Injury

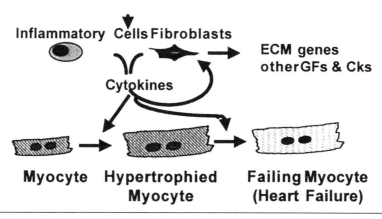

Fig. 1. *The 'cytokine hypothesis' of myocardial dysfunction.*

et al. used human atrial trabeculae obtained at the time of cardiac surgery, and measured developed force under control and IL-1 treated conditions. These investigators found that this cytokine depressed human myocardial function in a dose-dependent fashion and that this effect was synergistic with that of TNFα [20]. Recently we have investigated the expression of IL-1 mRNA in tissue and cells isolated from the explanted hearts of patients undergoing cardiac transplantation. These results are shown in Figure 2 and, confirming experimental data from both our lab and others, indicate that it is the non-muscle cell fraction largely responsible for IL-1 expression in these failing hearts.

IL-1 in animal models of myocardial dysfunction

In support of its role in the pathogenesis of human myocardial dysfunction, there have also been a number of reports on IL-1 expression using several animal models (both large and small) of myocardial dysfunction, including post-infarction, post-transplantation, and post-viral myocarditis. All of these investigations have shown that myocardial cells themselves are the source of IL-1 [21–27]. Additional work by our group using *ex vivo* material has found that the cardiac fibroblast is a source of IL-1. Specifically, while investigating the response of rat myocardial cells to episodes of experimental hypoxia/ischemia, we have found that the fibroblast expression of IL-1 increases substantially following brief episodes of hypoxic medium (neonatal cells), low flow ischemia-reperfusion (adult cells), and in the days to

weeks following myocardial infarction (adult cells, *in vivo*) [21,28] (Fig. 3). This is a highly cell-specific response in that IL-1 was not induced in the myocyte fractions of either age group under any experimental conditions.

Further, following the initial report by Hosenpud [29], several investigators have confirmed a negative inotropic/chronotropic effect for IL-1 using both whole heart and isolated cell preparations [30–32], suggesting that local expression may result in local effects.

Therapeutic responses to heart failure treatment may be associated with changes in IL-1 expression

Cause and effect is often difficult to prove with certainty in human studies. Although the observation that cytokine levels decrease in response to therapeutic maneuvers previously reported to improve overall myocardial prognosis (such as ACE inhibition and beta blockade) does not necessarily result from a true cause-effect relationship, this finding is consistent with benefit which may be directly related to an overall decrease in cytokine expression/effect [33,34]. Similar observations have also been recently reported in an animal model of heart failure treated with β-blockade [26]. In one recently published trial, cytokine levels were found to be reduced in a small series of LVAD-unloaded heart failure patients [35]. Further, therapies that have directly targeted either cytokines or their interaction with receptor have been associated with beneficial responses and outcomes [27,36,37].

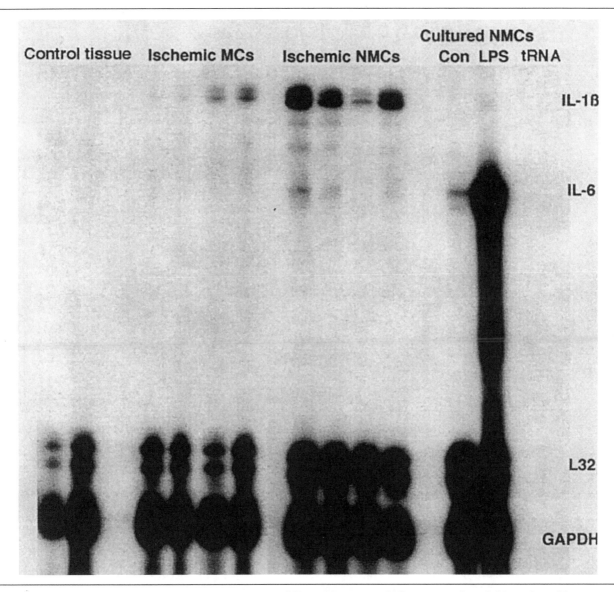

Fig. 2. *Failing human cardiac nonmyocytes are a source of IL-1β. Myocytes and Nonmyocytes from feshly explanted human ventricle were isolated by differential centrifugation and RNA isolated. Ten (10) micrograms were subjected to RNAse Protection with the human cytokine probe set from Pharmingen (Hck-2) followed by separation on a denaturing acrylamide gel. RNA samples identified as 'control' in this RPA are from tissue rather than isolated cells. As noted on the left, additional nonmyocytes were placed in culture and treated with endotoxin for 48 h as a positive control for inducible expression.*

Effectors of the IL-1 response: NO or not NO?, that is the question

IL-1 has been reported to signal through a wide variety of second messengers. The involvement of the nitric oxide system is particularly attractive as a possible means of cytokine-induced myocardial depression since NO has been described as a potent direct myocardial depressant, and iNOS is up-regulated in the failing heart [38–40]. Further, there have been a number of reports suggesting that ischemia-reperfusion, endotoxin and IL-1-induced myocardial depression *in vivo* is prevented by inhibition of the nitric oxide

synthase enzyme system [32,41,42], (reviewed in [43]). Similar *in vitro* experiments using cultured myocardial cells (both myocytes and non-myocytes) have likewise shown that IL-1 induces expression of the inducible form of nitric oxide (iNOS) at both mRNA and protein levels [8,10,44–46]. Concerning the mechanism of the increase in iNOS gene expression by IL-1, work by LaPointe et al. indicates that IL-1 induction of iNOS synthesis depends on both the p42/44 and p38 signaling pathways, acting primarily at the level of transcriptional regulation. A similar second messenger system is seen with the IL-1 activation of the brain natriuretic

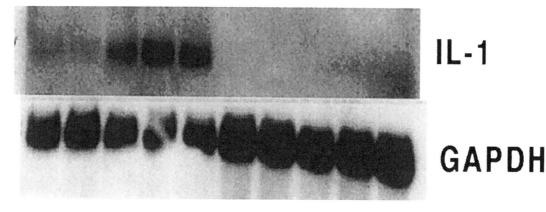

A   **Nonmyocyte   Myocyte**
     Con   Isch   Con   Isch

IL-1

GAPDH

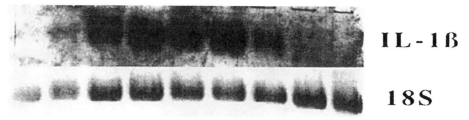

B   **hours   0 .5 2   6 12 24 48 72 72Con**

IL-1ß

18S

Fig. 3. *Cardiac nonmyocytes produce IL-1β.* **A.** *Adult rat hearts (Langendorff, non-working preparation) were subjected to a 30 min period of low flow ischemia followed by 30 min of reperfusion. Control adult cells were obtained by digestion after 60 min of continuous perfusion. Northern blots were sequentially probed with antisense riboprobes to mouse IL-1β and GAPDH RNAs.* **B.** *Cultures of neonatal rat cardiac fibroblasts were exposed to a 1% O$_2$ environment for the indicated times and total RNA harvested. Northern blots were sequentially probed with antisense riboprobes to mouse IL-1β and 18S RNAs.*

peptide (BNP) promoter [10,47]. BNP and other members of the natriuretic peptide family have *also* been implicated as effectors of cytokine-induced alterations in cardiac myocyte growth and gene expression [48–50] and, as such, represents an additional possible mechanism of IL-1 effects in the heart.

Additional second messengers have also been suggested to play a direct role in myocardial injury/dysfunction. For example, Oral et al. have implicated the sphingomyelinase pathway as responsible for TNF-induced repression [51]. This pathway is also activated by IL-1 (reviewed in [52]).

IL-1 and myocardial apoptosis

Apoptosis, the process of programmed cell death, has been implicated as a potential 'player' in the process of myocardial dysfunction (reviewed in [53]). Although this hypothesis is controversial,

the known connection between cytokines and apoptosis in other cell types makes the discussion of IL-1 and apoptosis germane to this review. Perhaps most pertinent is the suggestion that NO is the proximate mechanism of apoptosis. In this regard, Ing et al. recently reported that neonatal cardiac myocytes treated with a combination of the macrophage-derived cytokines IL-1, TNF?, and IFN?, exhibited a time-dependent induction of cardiac myocyte apoptosis, but not necrosis [54]. Although this effect required nearly 72 h to become manifest, it appeared to be due to oxygen free radicals and alterations in the cellular balance of Bak and Bcl-x. Similar findings were reported for both neonatal and adult rat ventricular myocytes by others and indicate an important role for free radicals, NO, the bcl-2 family, and p53 [55,56]. It should be noted that all of these investigations have been performed in relatively high density cultures and does not rule out the possibility that the delay in the observed effects is due to the paracrine release of pro-apoptotic substances by contaminating non-myocytes.

IL-1, calcium, and arrhythmogenesis

Many cardiac diseases in which cytokines are elevated are associated with an increased incidence of arrhythmias. Specifically, ventricular arrhythmias occur frequently in ischemia-reperfusion, hypertrophy and heart failure [57,58]. Moreover, it is apparent that the largest single cause of death in patients with dilated cardio-myopathy is, in fact, due to ventricular arrhythmia [59]. The presence of increased cytokines in patient populations exhibiting an increase in lethal arrhythmias has suggested the possibility that a direct relationship may exist.

Triggered activity, defined as repetitive activity in cardiac tissue arising from afterdepolarizations, has been implicated in the pathogenesis of both atrial tachycardias and ventricular tachyarrhythmias associated with ventricular hypertrophy and ischemia [60,61]. Afterdepolarizations are oscillations in the membrane potential and may occur early, before complete repolarization of the preceding action potential (EAD) or delayed, after complete repolarization (DAD). The amplitude of these afterdepolarizations can be subthreshold (i.e. not initiating a subsequent action potential) or they may reach threshold and repetitively induce action potentials resulting in sustained arrhythmias. The underlying pathophysiologic mechanism for this activity is not well elucidated, although elevated cytoplasmic calcium levels have been implicated [61,62]. Elevated levels of cytosolic calcium have also been implicated as contributing to the arrhythmogenic substrate in ischemic-myocardium [63].

In neonatal rat myocytes, SERCA 2A (the sarcoplasmic reticulum calcium-ATPase), phospholamban (a protein that modulates SERCA) as well as the voltage-gated calcium channel and calcium release channel are all decreased in response to IL-1 [4–7]. Consistent with these changes, intracellular calcium content has been reported to be abnormal in cytokine treated cardiac myocytes [64,65]. As such, the substrate for arrhythmogenesis in response to cytokines like IL-1 would seemingly be present in the failing heart.

IL-1 and myocardial protection

Although the data described to this point has suggested a primarily negative role for IL-1 and the heart, there have been some reports indicating a 'cardio-protective' role for cytokines like IL-1. Specifically, several investigators have found that IL-1 pre-treatment reduced myocardial injury in an ischemia-reperfusion model, an effect that was also seen with TNFα and felt to relate to the induction of the superoxide dismutase pathway of free-radical scavengers [66–69].

Finally, recent research from the Mann group found that myocardial infarctions performed in a background of genetic loss of both the type I and type II TNF receptors were larger than that of wild-type animals suggesting that this cytokine might play a protective role in the myocardial response to injury [70]. Although this has not yet been reported for IL-1, this, along with the above reports represent a precedent for a possible protective role for both of these cytokines in the heart and require a re-evaluation of the concept that cytokine expression is *always* maladaptive in the heart.

Unique nature of the IL-1 induced myocardial phenotype: studies with a cell culture model

In an effort to understand the potential influence of IL-1 in the heart, recombinant IL-1 has been administered to freshly isolated cultures of neonatal rat myocardial cells. These investigations indicate that IL-1β has novel effects on cardiac myocyte gene expression that contrasts with that seen with most hypertrophic agents such as the alpha$_1$-agonist phenylephrine. Specifically, IL-1 appears to induce a unique form of cardiac myocyte hypertrophy which is characterized by an increase in cell size with a net decrease in myofibrillar proteins, a form of hypertrophy that is reminiscent of pathological myocyte hypertrophy observed in the failing human heart [71,72]. Further, as indicated below, the electrophysiologic properties of the IL-1 treated myocyte are also similar to that seen in the failing heart. What has remained poorly understood are the mechanisms by which IL-1 alters the overall transcriptional program of the cardiac myocyte towards this pathologic state.

Conceptually, the difference between the physiologic and pathologic hypertrophy is likely to result from a fundamental difference in the action of the causative agents on factors involved in the induction of cell-specific gene products. Specifically, the classic hypertrophic phenotype is associated with an increase in the activity of transcription factors involved in stimulating the expression of these genes [73,75]. Conversely, IL-1 represses the action of agonists normally associated with the activation of myocyte-specific gene expression, an effect that appears to co-localize with the activity of several negative transcriptional regulators [5,76].

IL-1 represses induction of the pathologic gene program

Our initial work indicated that IL-1 did not activate, and may even repress, two of the fetal program genes (skeletal actin and βMHC) under basal conditions. It was unclear, however, whether this repression extended to situations where these genes were up-regulated. In our initial investigations, myocytes were treated with the alpha$_1$-agonist phenylephrine and IL-1 at the physiologically relevant concentrations known to induce maximal changes in the induction of skeletal actin and βMHC in total cell protein. Although there was no additive (or repressive) effect on either total protein or total RNA during co-treatment, IL-1 prevented the increase in mRNAs for both genes normally seen with phenylephrine. Transient transfection of myocytes with plasmids containing promoter elements for the skeletal actin and β myosin heavy chain genes confirmed that the negative IL-1 effect resulted from action at the transcriptional level and localized this response to specific regions of the two promoters [5].

IL-1 represses T₃-mediated changes in myocyte gene expression

Work by a number of laboratories indicates that cardiac myocytes respond to thyroid hormone, both *in vivo* and *in vitro*, by inducing SERCA 2a [77], skeletal α-actin [78,79], and α-MHC gene expression, while repressing β-MHC [78,79]. To investigate whether, in addition to its effects on adrenergic stimulation, IL-1 also alters the expression of T₃-inducible genes, we evaluated the mRNA expression of skeletal α-actin and SERCA 2a after treatment with IL-1, T₃, both, or neither. Although both genes are induced in the presence of 20 ng/ml T₃, co-treatment with IL-1 repressed T₃-mediated induction of SERCA and skeletal α-actin mRNA expression and reversed the T₃ effects on *both* MHC-isogenes [80].

IL-1 prolongs myocyte action potential and induces triggered activity

To determine the electrophysiological effects of IL-1, primary cultures of neonatal rat cardiac myocytes were treated with IL-1 for 48 h and electrophysiologic studies performed [81]. These investigations indicate that treatment with IL-1 significantly prolonged action potential duration (161.0 ± 76.8 ms vs. 106.6 ± 72.6 ms) and decreased action potential amplitude (133.9 ± 15.7 mV vs 147.4 ± 17.3 mV).

As noted previously, triggered activity may be one mechanism of arrhythmogenesis in the heart. As such, the finding of an increase of this activity in IL-1 treated cells would provide support for a potential cause-effect relationship between increased cytokines and arrhythmia in heart failure patients. As indicated in Figure 4, although no triggered activity can be induced in control cells, IL-1 induces both subthreshold DADs and triggered action potentials. Further, when Ryanodine was added to the external, no triggered activity was induced, even when the external Ca^{2+} concentration was increased to 10 mM, implicating the release of calcium by the sacro-

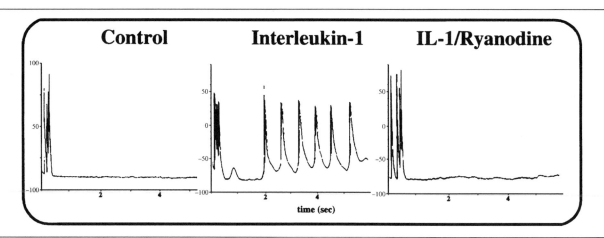

Fig. 4. *IL-1β-induced triggered activity in neonatal rat cardiocytes is blocked by ryanodine. Myocytes in serum-free medium were treated for 48 h with IL-1β (1 ng/ml) and subjected to electrophysiologic testing. Following patching of the cell, action potentials were evoked with a 2 ms depolarizing current pulse at 0.2 Hz in the current-clamp mode. The following pacing protocol was performed: a basic drive train of eight, 2 ms current pulses was repeated at cycle lengths of 500, 400, 300, 200 and 100 ms. Following each train, 4 extra pulses were applied, decrementing by 100 ms for the 500, 400 and 300 trains, by 50 ms for the 200 ms train, and by 25 ms for the 100 ms train. DADs and triggered activity were then recorded for the next 5 s.*

plasmic reticulum in the arrhythmogenic effects of IL-1.

IL-1 signaling and associated transcription factors

As is the case for most cytokines, the biological action of IL-1 is mediated through the dimerization of specific cell surface reporters. In contrast to many agonists, however, IL-1 binding leads to the activation of a variety of signaling pathways, including sphingomyelinase, protein kinase C, stress-activated protein kinases, and activation of tyrosine kinases even though the IL-1 receptor complex does not contain sequences typical of a tyrosine kinase domain (reviewed in [82]).

These different pathways ultimately result in a change in cellular gene expression through their action on several downstream transcription factors. Perhaps the best studied of these are the increases in NFκB and AP-1 translocation. Although there has been little work done on the induction of transcription factors in myocardial cells following IL-1 treatment, both NFκB and AP-1 binding activity increases in response to IL-1 (Fig. 5) and have been implicated by both our lab and others in the stimulation of inducible nitric oxide and adhesion molecule expression (ICAM-1 and VCAM-1 [8,9]).

IL-1 inhibits thyroid hormone effects on the alpha myosin heavy chain gene via the AP-1 transcription factor

As noted previously, IL-1 represses basal expression of the adult myosin heavy chain isoform (αMHC) and antagonizes the stimulatory effects of thyroid hormone. Transient transfections with the αMHC promoter has further supported our observation that IL-1 action on the αMHC gene product is transcriptional in nature and appeared to require the presence of the thyroid hormone response element(s) (TREs). The transcription factor AP-1, which is comprised of either a cjun/cfos heterodimer or a cjun homodimer is known to interact with members of the nuclear receptor family, such as the T3-receptor, by protein–protein interaction (reviewed in [83]). It also modifies nuclear receptor mediated transcriptional activation in several genes [84]. Furthermore, IL-1 has been reported to increase AP-1 DNA binding activity in several cell types including cardiac myocytes [8,9,85], making it a potential effector of IL-1 activity in our cells.

Two additional cytokine-responsive transcriptional regulators have also been described and may play an important role in the effects of IL-1 in the heart. Specifically, a 'cardiac-specific ankyrin repeat protein' that has important effects on the regulation of myocyte-specific gene expression has been reported [86]. Called 'CARP', this

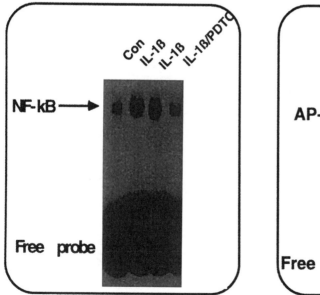
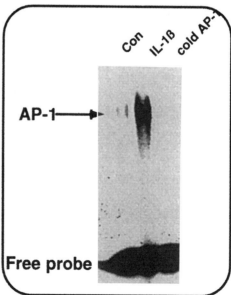

Fig. 5. *IL-1β induced NFκB and AP-1 binding activity in cardiac myocytes. Neonatal rat cardiac myocytes were treated for 48 h with IL-1β (1 ng/ml) followed by nuclear extract preparation. Equivalent amount of protein (~5 μg) were incubated with ³²P-labeled factor-specific oligo-nucleotides and separated by non-denaturing electrophoresis. Specificity was shown for both by the inclusion of an excess of unlabeled oligo (shown here for AP-1 only). Of note was the decrease in NFκB binding following treatment with the anti-oxidant PDTC, previously suggested to decrease NFκB activation in other cell types.*

factor is also known as the 'cardiac adriamycin-responsive protein' [87]. It is noteworthy that this transcription factor does not appear to be, in fact, cardiac-specific and was previously described by Chu et al. as a cytokine responsive ankyrin repeat protein, C-193 [88]. Chu reported that this protein was induced in response to both IL-1 and TNF in an inflammatory cell background and suggested that it played an important regulatory role in cytokine responsive tissues/cells, although the target(s) were not known at that time. In the heart, the co-localization of the activity of this protein with the HF-1a element and its ability to co-repress the activity of the myosin light chain 2 promoter in cardiac muscle cells is suggestive of an important regulatory role in myocardium [86]. Further, this factor is downstream of the well described cardiac-specific transcriptional regulator Nkx [89,90].

IL-1 inhibition of myosin light chain 2v expression co-localizes with the CARP binding site (HF-1a)

Preliminary work in our laboratory has extended the repressive effects of IL-1 to an additional

contractile protein gene, MLC-2v. Shown by others to be induced by adrenergic stimulation in a manner similar to that of the skeletal actin and βMHC genes, the elements responsible for MLC-2v induction have been reported to be due to the action of both ubiquitous (YB-1) and tissue-specific transcriptional regulators (MEF-2, HF-1b) [91,92]. In order to see if the repressive effect of IL-1 extended to this contractile protein as well, we performed a series of experiments with the promoter elements shown to be important in the regulation of this gene in cardiac myocytes. As shown in Figure 6, IL-1 down-regulated expression of the MLC-2v constructs and appeared to co-localize with the HF-1a element. Previous work by the Chien laboratory has suggested that this area of the MLC-2v promoter may be negatively regulated by CARP [86,93].

In addition to CARP, the involvement of the bifunctional regulator yin yang-1 (YY1) in modulating the expression of several muscle-specific genes has been known for some time [73,94–96]. Our previous work which localized the IL-1 effect to specific promoter sequences in the skeletal actin and β-myosin heavy chain genes was noteworthy since these fragments included serum response elements containing consensus sites

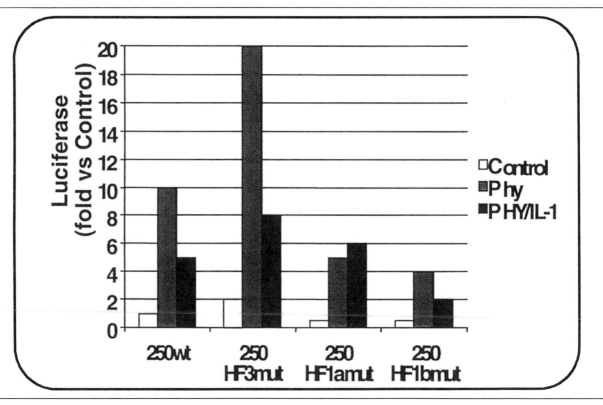

Fig. 6. *IL-1β repression of MLC-2v promoter activity co-localizes with the HF-1a element. Cardiac myocyctes were transfected with a series of MLC-2v luciferase promoter:reporter constructs and the cells treated with or without IL-1β (1 ng/ml) for 48 h. Luciferase activity was normalized for transfection efficiency and expressed as a ratio of treated to control for all constructs.*

for YY1 [5]. The overall importance of YY1 was confirmed in subsequent experiments, finding that the IL-1 effects are lost when these sites are mutated [5,76]. In addition, we recently reported that IL-1 alters both the abundance, phosphorylation state, and DNA binding activity for YY1 [76].

YY1 protein levels are increased in failing human and rat ventricular myocytes

All of the preliminary data shown above on the effect of IL-1 on cardiac myocyte growth/gene expression and co-localization with specific nuclear effector molecules has been accomplished using primary cultures obtained from neonatal rat hearts. In an effort to confirm the relevance the cell culture findings, myocyte proteins have been obtained from a series of experimental animals 2 weeks after left coronary occlusion as well as from 4 individual human hearts undergoing primary cardiac transplantation. As indicated in Figure 7, YY1 protein is increased in all of the specimens from the injured hearts, but not from control (or sham) specimens. Similarly, an increase in the 35 Kd unprocessed pro-IL-1 protein (i.e. pre-interleukin-1 converting enzyme cleavage) is seen in the whole heart tissue from a

patient with dilated cardiomyopathy but not in the extracts from isolated cardiac myocytes from two patients with ischemic cardiomyopathy. This would be expected if most of the IL-1 production in response to injury comes, in fact, from the non-muscle cells of the heart. It is noteworthy that the increases in pro-IL-1β are reflected by an increase in iNOS activity in the same samples, consistent with the effect of local IL-1 production.

IL-1 does not induce a generalized decrease in gene transcription

Although the data described above suggests that IL-1 might induce a generalized decrease in myocyte RNA polymerase II activity, investigations of several genes indicate that this is not the case. Specifically, IL-1 treatment increases the myocyte expression of both c-fos and c-myc proto-oncogenes as well as the housekeeping β-actin gene, and fails to blunt the phenylephrine response on β-actin promoter induction [5]. Further, cardiac myocytes respond to IL-1 stimulation with an increase in both the inducible form of nitric oxide synthase (iNOS) and the cellular adhesion molecules ICAM-1 and VCAM-1 [8,9]. Taken together, these results suggest that, rather than causing a generalized decrease in myocyte

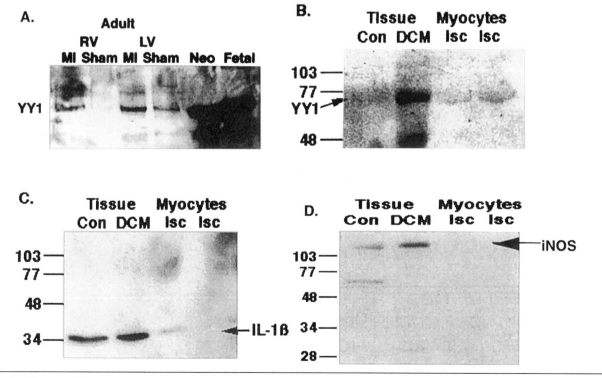

Fig. 7. *IL-1β and YY1 expression are increased in failing hearts. Panel* **A** *represents YY1 expression obtained from myocytes isolated 2 weeks following left coronary occlusion in the rat. Panels* **B**, **C** *and* **D** *are from human hearts extracted either as whole tissue (Control and DCM) or from myocytes isolated following collagenase perfusion and gradient centrifugation (Isc).*

mRNA transcription, IL-1 induces a selective decrease in the expression of *myocyte-specific* gene products.

Conclusions

The overall hypothesis of the investigations described in this review and others in this issue is that cytokines play a critical role in the progression of the failing heart and that therapies aimed at altering either cytokine expression or effects will be beneficial. The attractive nature of such an immunomodulatory approach to the failing heart is its potential ability to complement the presently existing therapeutic armamentarium rather than serving as 'just another ACE inhibitor.' Specifically, such an agent or agents would be used in conjunction with standard therapies with an expectation that additional benefit(s) would be realized.

The data described above has confirmed that one of these pro-inflammatory cytokines, IL-1, induces a unique hypertropic phenotype. Specifically, IL-1 treated myocytes dramatically down-regulate expression of a variety of myocyte-specific genes including those involved in calcium handling. This occurs simultaneously with an up-regulation of markers of inflammation such as nitric oxide and adhesion molecules and appears to involve the activity of a specific set of negative regulatory transcription factors. As a reflection of the abnormalities of calcium homeostasis, the IL-1 treated myocyte also has an abnormal action potential duration and a lower threshold for the induction of triggered activity. All of these features (i.e. a hypertrophic myocyte with diminished myofibrillar content, abnormal calcium handling, and a propensity to 'arrhythmia') are similar to those seen in the end-stage and failing heart, a clinical circumstance that is also associated with an increase in the expression of pro-inflammatory cytokines. As partial proof of concept, preliminary data gathered in human heart failure specimens suggests that alterations in myocardial cytokine expression are common to those seen in animal models. These findings serve to validate the cytokine hypothesis and emphasize the need to pursue the mechanisms of cytokine-induced alterations in gene program as a potentially novel approach to clinical myocardial dysfunction.

Acknowledgments

This work was supported by grants to CSL from the NIH (HL58974 and HL59428). I thank Drs. Monica Patten, Weizhong Wang, Rachid Kacimi, James Palmer, Javier Lopez, Shadi Aminololama-Shakeri, and Jodi Rosenbleet, the research fellows who have contributed to this work. Without their dedication, none of these investigations would have been possible.

References

1. Mauviel A. Cytokine regulation of metalloproteinase gene expression. *J Cell Biochem* 1993;53:288–295.
2. Booz GW, Baker KM. Molecular signalling mechanisms controlling growth and function of cardiac fibroblasts. *Cardiovasc Res* 1995;30:537–543.
3. Li YY, McTiernan CF, Feldman AM. Proinflammatory cytokines regulate tissue inhibitors of metalloproteinases and disintegrin metalloproteinase in cardiac cells. *Cardiovasc Res* 1999;42:162–172.
4. Palmer JN, Hartogensis WE, Patten M, Fortuin FD, Long CS. Interleukin-1 beta induces cardiac myocyte growth but inhibits cardiac fibroblast proliferation in culture. *J Clin Invest* 1995;95:2555–2564.
5. Patten M, Hartogensis WE, Long CS. IL-1β is a negative regulator of α1-adrenergic induced cardiac gene expression. *J Biol Chem* 1996;271:21134–21141.
6. Thaik CM, Calderone A, Takahashi N, Colucci WS. Interleukin-1 beta modulates the growth and phenotype of neonatal rat cardiac myocytes. *J Clin Invest* 1995;96:1093–1099.
7. McTiernan CF, Lemster BH, Frye C, Brooks S, Combes A, Feldman AM. Interleukin-1 beta inhibits phospholamban gene expression in cultured cardiomyocytes. *Circ Res* 1997;81:493–503.
8. Kacimi R, Long CS, Karliner JS. Chronic hypoxia modulates the interleukin-1beta-stimulated inducible nitric oxide synthase pathway in cardiac myocytes. *Circulation* 1997;96:1937–1943.
9. Kacimi R, Karliner JS, Koudssi F, Long CS. Expression and regulation of adhesion molecules in cardiac cells by cytokines. *Circ Res* 1998;82:576–586.
10. LaPointe MC, Isenovic E. Interleukin-1beta regulation of inducible nitric oxide synthase and cyclooxygenase-2 involves the p42/44 and p38 MAPK signaling pathways in cardiac myocytes. *Hypertension* 1999;33:276–282.
11. Han R, Ray P, Baughman K, Feldman A. Detection of interleukin and inteleukin-receptor mRNA in human heart by polymerase chain reaction. *Biochem Biophys Res Comm* 1991;181:520–523.
12. Francis SE, Holden H, Holt CM, Duff GW. Interleukin-1 in myocardium and coronary arteries of patients with dilated cardiomyopathy. *J Mol Cell Cardiol* 1998;30:215–223.
13. Satoh M, Tamura G, Segawa I, Tashiro A, Hiramori K, Satodate R. Expression of cytokine genes and presence of enteroviral genomic RNA in endomyocardial biopsy tissues of myocarditis and dilated cardiomyopathy. *Virchows Arch* 1996;427:503–509.
14. Matsumori A, Yamada T, Suzuki H, Matoba Y, Sasayama S. Increased circulating cytokines in patients with myocarditis and cardiomyopathy. *Br Heart J* 1994;72:561–566.
15. Guillen I, Blanes M, Gomez-Lechon M-J, Castell JV. Cytokine signaling during myocardial infarction: sequential appearance of IL-1β and IL-6. *Am J Physiol* 1995;269:R229–R235.

16. Lagoo AS, George JF, Naftel DC, Griffin AK, Kirklin JK, Lagoo DS, Hardy KJ, Savunen T, McGiffin DC. Semiquantitative measurement of cytokine messenger RNA in endomyocardium and peripheral blood mononuclear cells from human heart transplant recipients. *J Heart Lung Transplant* 1996;15:206–217.

17. Kumar A, Thota V, Dee L, Olson J, Uretz E, Parrillo JE. Tumor necrosis factor alpha and interleukin 1beta are responsible for *in vitro* myocardial cell depression induced by human septic shock serum. *J Exp Med* 1996;183:949–958.

18. Testa M, Yeh M, Lee P, Fanelli R, Loperfido F, Berman JW, LeJemtel TH. Circulating levels of cytokines and their endogenous modulators in patients with mild to severe congestive heart failure due to coronary artery disease or hypertension. *J Am Coll Cardiol* 1996;28:964–971.

19. Yegin O, Coskun M, Ertug H. Cytokines in acute rheumatic fever. *Eur J Pediatr* 1997;156:25–29.

20. Cain BS, Meldrum DR, Dinarello CA, Meng X, Joo KS, Banerjee A, Harken AH. Tumor necrosis factor-alpha and interleukin-1beta synergistically depress human myocardial function [see comments]. *Critical Care Medicine* 1999;27:1309–1318.

21. Yue P, Massie BM, Simpson PC, Long CS. Cytokine expression increases in nonmyocytes from rats with postinfarction heart failure. *Am J Physiol* 1998;275:H250–H258.

22. Ono K, Matsumori A, Shioi T, Furukawa Y, Sasayama S. Cytokine gene expression after myocardial infarction in rat hearts: possible implication in left ventricular remodeling. *Circulation* 1998;98:149–156.

23. Shioi T, Matsumori A, Kihara Y, Inoko M, Ono K, Iwanaga Y, Yamada T, Iwasaki A, Matsushima K, Sasayama S. Increased expression of interleukin-1β and monocyte chemotactic and activating factor/monocyte chemoattracting protein-1 in the hypertrophied and failing heart with pressure overload. *Circ Res* 1997;81:664–671.

24. Chandrasekar B, Melby PC, Troyer DA, Colston JT, Freeman GL. Temporal expression of pro-inflammatory cytokines and inducible nitric oxide synthase in experimental acute Chagasic cardiomyopathy. *Am J Pathol* 1998;152:925–934.

25. Freeman GL, Colston JT, Zabalgoitia M, Chandrasekar B. Contractile depression and expression of proinflammatory cytokines and iNOS in viral myocarditis. *Am J Physiol* 1998;274:H249–258.

26. Prabhu SD, Chandrasekar B, Murray DR, Freeman GL. beta-adrenergic blockade in developing heart failure: effects on myocardial inflammatory cytokines, nitric oxide, and remodeling. *Circulation* 2000;101:2103–2109.

27. Kubota T, Bounoutas GS, Miyagishima M, Kadokami T, Sanders VJ, Bruton C, Robbins PD, McTiernan CF, Feldman AM. Soluble tumor necrosis factor receptor abrogates myocardial inflammation but not hypertrophy in cytokine-induced cardiomyopathy [In Process Citation]. *Circulation* 2000;101:2518–2525.

28. Long CS, Palmer JN, Hartogensis W, Honbo N, Miguel T, Grunfeld C, Karliner JS. Hypoxia stimulates interleukin-1 RNA expression by cardiac non-myocytes in culture. *Clin Res* 1993;41:145A (abstract).

29. Hosenpud J, Campbell S, Mendelson D. Interleukin-1-induced myocardial depression in an isolated beating heart preparation. *J Heart Transplant* 1989;8:460–464.

30. Weissensee D, Bereiter-Hahn J, Schoeppe W, Löw-Friedrich I. Effects of cytokines on the contractility of cultured cardiac myocytes. *Int J Immunopharmac* 1993;15:581–587.

31. Evans HG, Lewis MJ, Shah AM. Interleukin-1 beta modulates myocardial contraction via dexamethasone sensitive production of nitric oxide [see comments]. *Cardiovasc Res* 1993;27:1486–1490.

32. Oyama J, Shimokawa H, Momii H, Cheng X, Fukuyama N, Arai Y, Egashira K, Nakazawa H, Takeshita A. Role of nitric oxide and peroxynitrite in the cytokine-induced sustained myocardial dysfunction in dogs *in vivo*. *J Clin Invest* 1998;101:2207–2214.

33. Gullestad L, Aukrust P, Ueland T, Espevik T, Yee G, Vagelos R, Froland SS, Fowler M. Effect of high- versus low-dose angiotensin converting enzyme inhibition on cytokine levels in chronic heart failure [see comments]. *J Am Coll Cardiol* 1999;34:2061–2067.

34. Matsumori A, Ono K, Nishio R, Nose Y, Sasayama S. Amlodipine inhibits the production of cytokines induced by ouabain. *Cytokine* 2000;12:294–297.

35. Torre-Amione G, Stetson SJ, Youker KA, Durand JB, Radovancevic B, Delgado RM, Frazier OH, Entman ML, Noon GP. Decreased expression of tumor necrosis factor-alpha in failing human myocardium after mechanical circulatory support: A potential mechanism for cardiac recovery. *Circulation* 1999;100:1189–1193.

36. Kapadia S, Torre-Amione G, Yokoyama T, Mann DL. Soluble TNF binding proteins modulate the negative inotropic properties of TNF-alpha *in vitro*. *Am J Physiol* 1995;268:H517–H525.

37. Deswal A, Seta Y, Bozkurt B, Parilti-Eiswirth S, Hayes A, Blosch CM, Mann DL. Safety and Efficacy of a Soluble P75 Tumor necrosis factor receptor (Enbrel, Etanercept) in patients with advanced heart failure. *Circulation* 1999;99:3224–3226.

38. de Belder AJ, Radomski MW, Why HJ, Richardson PJ, Martin JF. Myocardial calcium-independent nitric oxide synthase activity is present in dilated cardiomyopathy, myocarditis, and postpartum cardiomyopathy but not in ischaemic or valvar heart disease. *Br Heart J* 1995;74:426–430.

39. Habib FM, Springall DR, Davies GJ, Oakley CM, Yacoub MH, Polak JM. Tumour necrosis factor and inducible nitric oxide synthase in dilated cardiomyopathy [see comments]. *Lancet* 1996;347:1151–1155.

40. Haywood GA, Tsao PS, von der Leyen HE, Mann MJ, Keeling PJ, Trindade PT, Lewis NP, Byrne CD, Rickenbacher PR, Bishopric NH, Cooke JP, McKenna WJ, Fowler MB. Expression of inducible nitric oxide synthase in human heart failure. *Circulation* 1996;93:1087–1094.

41. Roberts AB, Vodovotz Y, Roche NS, Sporn MB, Nathan CF. Role of nitric oxide in antagonistic effects of transforming growth factor-beta and interleukin-

1beta on the beating rate of cultured cardiac myocytes. *Mol Endocrinol* 1992;6:1921–1930.

42. Keaney JF, Jr, Hare JM, Balligand JL, Loscalzo J, Smith TW, Colucci WS. Inhibition of nitric oxide synthase augments myocardial contractile responses to beta-adrenergic stimulation. *Am J Physiol* 1996;271:H2646–H2652.

43. Kojda G, Kottenberg K. Regulation of basal myocardial function by NO. *Cardiovasc Res* 1999;41:514–523.

44. Tsujino M, Hirata Y, Imai T, Kanno K, Eguchi S, Ito H, Marumo F. Induction of nitric oxide synthase gene by interleukin-1 beta in cultured rat cardiocytes. *Circulation* 1994;90:375–383.

45. Balligand JL, Ungureanu-Longrois D, Simmons WW, Pimental D, Malinski TA, Kapturczak M, Taha Z, Lowenstein CJ, Davidoff AJ, Kelly RA, et al.. Cytokine-inductible nitric oxide synthase (iNOS) expression in cardiac myocytes. Characterization and regulation of iNOS expression and detection of iNOS activity in single cardiac myocytes *in vitro*. *J Biol Chem* 1994;269:27580–27588.

46. LaPointe MC, Sitkins JR. Mechanisms of interleukin-1beta regulation of nitric oxide synthase in cardiac myocytes. *Hypertension* 1996;27:709–714.

47. He Q, LaPointe MC. Interleukin-1beta regulation of the human brain natriuretic peptide promoter involves Ras-, Rac-, and p38 kinase-dependent pathways in cardiac myocytes. *Hypertension* 1999;33:283–289.

48. Bezie Y, Mesnard L, Longrois D, Samson F, Perret C, Mercadier JJ, Laurent S. Interactions between endothelin-1 and atrial natriuretic peptide influence cultured chick cardiac myocyte contractility. *Eur J Pharmacol* 1996;311:241–248.

49. Wu CF, Bishopric NH, Pratt RE. Atrial natriuretic peptide induces apoptosis in neonatal rat cardiac myocytes. *J Biol Chem* 1997;272:14860–14866.

50. Horio T, Nishikimi T, Yoshihara F, Matsuo H, Takishita S, Kangawa K. Inhibitory regulation of hypertrophy by endogenous atrial natriuretic peptide in cultured cardiac myocytes. *Hypertension* 2000;35:19–24.

51. Oral H, Dorn GW, 2nd, Mann DL. Sphingosine mediates the immediate negative inotropic effects of tumor necrosis factor-alpha in the adult mammalian cardiac myocyte. *J Biol Chem* 1997;272:4836–4842.

52. Kuno K, Matsushima K. The IL-1 receptor signaling pathway. *J Leukoc Biol* 1994;56:542–547.

53. Kang PM, Izumo S. Apoptosis and heart failure: A critical review of the literature. *Circ Res* 2000;86:1107–1113.

54. Ing DJ, Zang J, Dzau VJ, Webster KA, Bishopric NH. Modulation of cytokine-induced cardiac myocyte apoptosis by nitric oxide, Bak, and Bcl-x. *Circ Res* 1999;84:21–33.

55. Arstall MA, Sawyer DB, Fukazawa R, Kelly RA. Cytokine-mediated apoptosis in cardiac myocytes: the role of inducible nitric oxide synthase induction and peroxynitrite generation [see comments]. *Circ Res* 1999;85:829–840.

56. Pinsky DJ, Aji W, Szabolcs M, Athan ES, Liu Y, Yang YM, Kline RP, Olson KE, Cannon PJ. Nitric oxide triggers programmed cell death (apoptosis) of

adult rat ventricular myocytes in culture. *Am J Physiol* 1999;277:H1189–H1199.

57. Levy D, Anderson KM, Savage DD, Balkus SA, Kannel WB, Castelli WP. Risk of ventricular arrhythmias in left ventricular hypertrophy: the Framingham Heart Study. *Am J Cardiol* 1987;60:560–565.

58. Packer M. Sudden unexpected death in patients with congestive heart failure: a second frontier. *Circulation* 1985;72:681–685.

59. Kannel WB, Plehn JF, Cupples LA. Cardiac failure and sudden death in the Framingham Study. *Am Heart J* 1988;115:869–875.

60. Ferrier GR, Moffat MP, Lukas A. Possible mechanisms of ventricular arrhythmias elicited by ischemia followed by reperfusion. Studies on isolated canine ventricular tissues. *Circ Res* 1985;56:184–194.

61. Aronson RS. Afterpotentials and triggered activity in hypertrophied myocardium from rats with renal hypertension. *Circ Res* 1981;48:720–727.

62. Ming Z, Nordin C, Aronson RS. Role of L-type calcium channel window current in generating current-induced early afterdepolarizations. *J Cardiovasc Electrophysiol* 1994;5:323–334.

63. Dangman KH, Dresdner KJ, Zaim S. Automatic and triggered impulse initiation in canine subepicardial ventricular muscle cells from border zones of 24-hour transmural infarcts. New mechanisms for malignant cardiac arrhythmias? *Circulation* 1988;78:1020–1030.

64. Bick RJ, Liao JP, King TW, LeMaistre A, McMillin JB, Buja LM. Temporal effects of cytokines on neonatal cardiac myocyte Ca^{2+} transients and adenylate cyclase activity. *Am J Physiol* 1997;272:H1937–H1944.

65. Bick RJ, Wood DE, Poindexter B, McMillin JB, Karoly A, Wang D, Bunting R, McCann T, Law GJ, Buja LM. Cytokines increase neonatal cardiac myocyte calcium concentrations: the involvement of nitric oxide and cyclic nucleotides. *Journal of Interferon & Cytokine Research* 1999;19:645–653.

66. Brown J, White C, Terada L, Grosso M, Shanley P, Mulvin D, Banerjee A, Whitman G, Harken A, Repine J. Interleukin 1 pretreatment decreases ischemia/reperfusion injury. *Proc Natl Acad Sci (USA)* 1990;87:5026–5030.

67. Eddy L, Goeddel D, Wong G. Tumor necrosis factor-α pretreatment is protective in a rat model of myocardial ischemia-reperfusion injury. *Biochem Biophys Res Comm* 1992;184:1056–1059.

68. Maulik N, Engelman RM, Wei Z, Lu D, Rousou JA, Das DK. Interleukin-1 alpha preconditioning reduces myocardial ischemia reperfusion injury. *Circulation* 1993;88:II387–II394.

69. Nogae C, Makino N, Hata T, Nogae I, Takahashi S, Suzuki K, Taniguchi N, Yanaga T. Interleukin 1 alpha-induced expression of manganous superoxide dismutase reduces myocardial reperfusion injury in the rat. *J Mol Cell Cardiol* 1995;27:2091–2099.

70. Kurrelmeyer KM, Michael LH, Baumgarten G, Taffet GE, Peschon JJ, Sivasubramanian N, Entman ML, Mann DL. Endogenous tumor necrosis factor protects the adult cardiac myocyte against ischemic-induced apoptosis in a murine model of acute myocardial infarction. *Proc Natl Acad Sci US A* 2000;97:5456–5461.

71. Katagiri T, Kitsu T, Akiyama K, Takeyama Y, Niitani H. Alterations in fine structures of myofibrils and structural proteins in patients with dilated cardiomyopathy—studies with biopsied heart tissues. *Jpn Circ J* 1987;51:682–688.

72. Zimmer G, Zimmermann R, Hess OM, Schneider J, Kubler W, Krayenbuehl HP, Hagl S, Mall G. Decreased concentration of myofibrils and myofiber hypertrophy are structural determinants of impaired left ventricular function in patients with chronic heart diseases: a multiple logistic regression analysis. *J Am Coll Cardiol* 1992;20:1135–1142.

73. MacLellan WR, Lee TC, Schwartz RJ, Schneider MD. Transforming growth factor-beta response elements of the skeletal alpha-actin gene. Combinatorial action of serum response factor, YY1, and the SV40 enhancer-binding protein, TEF-1. *J Biol Chem* 1994;269:16754–16760.

74. Kariya K-I, Farrance IKG, Simpson PC. Transcriptional enhancer factor-1 in cardiac myocytes interacts with an α1-adrenergic- and β-protein kinase C-inducible element in the rat β-myosin heavy chain promoter. *J Biol Chem* 1993;268:26658–26662.

75. Karns LR, Kariya K, Simpson PC. M-CAT, CArG, and Sp1 elements are required for alpha 1-adrenergic induction of the skeletal alpha-actin promoter during cardiac myocyte hypertrophy. Transcriptional enhancer factor-1 and protein kinase C as conserved transducers of the fetal program in cardiac growth. *J Biol Chem* 1995;270:410–417.

76. Patten M, Wang W, Shakeri S, Burson M, Long CS. IL-1β increases YY1 abundance and DNA-binding activity in cultured cardiac myocytes. *J Mol Cell Cardiol* 2000;32:1341–1352.

77. Rohrer DK, Hartong R, Dillmann WH. Influence of thyroid hormone and retinoic acid on slow sarcoplasmic reticulum Ca^{2+} ATPase and myosin heavy chain alpha gene expression in cardiac myocytes. Delineation of cis-active DNA elements that confer responsiveness to thyroid hormone but not to retinoic acid. *J Biol Chem* 1991;266:8638–8646.

78. Collie ES, Muscat GE. The human skeletal alpha-actin promoter is regulated by thyroid hormone: identification of a thyroid hormone response element. *Cell Growth Differ* 1993;4:269–279.

79. Gustafson TA, Markham BE, Morkin E. Effects of thyroid hormone on alpha-actin and myosin heavy chain gene expression in cardiac and skeletal muscles of the rat: measurement of mRNA content using synthetic oligonucleotide probes. *Circ Res* 1986;59:194–201.

80. Patten M, Long CS. IL-1β blocks thyroid hormone regulation of alpha and beta myosin heavy chain. *Circulation* 1996;94:I-531.

81. Palma EC, Keung EC, Simpson PC, Long CS, Lee RJ. Cytokine-induced triggered activity in isolated neonatal rat myocytes: a new mechanism of arrhythmogenesis. *PACE* 1998;21:898 (abstract).

82. O'Neill LA, Greene C. Signal transduction pathways activated by the IL-1 receptor family: ancient signaling machinery in mammals, insects, and plants. *J Leukoc Biol* 1998;63:650–657.

83. Pfahl M. Nuclear Receptor/AP-1 interaction. *Endocrine Reviews* 1993;14:651–658.

84. Zhang X-K, Wills K, Husmann M, Herrmann T, Pfahl M. Novel pathway for thyroid hormone receptor action through interaction with jun and fos oncogene activities. *Mol Cell Biol* 1991;11:6016–6025.

85. Muegge K, Vila M, Gusella G, Musso T, Herrlich P, Stein B, Durum S. Interleukin 1 induction of the *c-jun* promoter. *Proc Natl Acad Sci USA* 1993;90:7054–7058.

86. Zou Y, Evans S, Chen J, Kuo HC, Harvey RP, Chien KR. CARP, a cardiac ankyrin repeat protein, is downstream in the Nkx2-5 homeobox gene pathway. *Development* 1997;124:793–804.

87. Jeyaseelan R, Poizat C, Baker RK, Abdishoo S, Isterabadi LB, Lyons GE, Kedes L. A novel cardiac-restricted target for doxorubicin. CARP, a nuclear modulator of gene expression in cardiac progenitor cells and cardiomyocytes. *J Biol Chem* 1997;272:22800–22808.

88. Chu W, Burns DK, Swerlick RA, Presky DH. Identification and characterization of a novel cytokine-inducible nuclear protein from human endothelial cells. *J Biol Chem* 1995;270:10236–10245.

89. Takimoto E, Mizuno T, Terasaki F, Shimoyama M, Honda H, Shiojima I, Hiroi Y, Oka T, Hayashi D, Hirai H, Kudoh S, Toko H, Kawamura K, Nagai R, Yazaki Y, Komuro I. Up-regulation of natriuretic peptides in the ventricle of Csx/Nkx2–5 transgenic mice. *Biochem Biophys Res Commun* 2000;270:1074–1079.

90. Kuo H, Chen J, Ruiz-Lozano P, Zou Y, Nemer M, Chien KR. Control of segmental expression of the cardiac-restricted ankyrin repeat protein gene by distinct regulatory pathways in murine cardiogenesis. *Development* 1991;126:4223–4234.

91. Zhu H, Garcia AV, Ross RS, Evans SM, Chien KR. A conserved 28-base-pair element (HF-1) in the rat cardiac myosin light-chain-2 gene confers cardiac-specific and alpha-adrenergic-inducible expression in cultured neonatal rat myocardial cells. *Mol Cell Biol* 1991;11:2273–2281.

92. Navankasattusas S, Zhu H, Garcia AV, Evans SM, Chien KR. A ubiquitous factor (HF-1a) and a distinct muscle factor (HF-1b/MEF-2) form an E-box-independent pathway for cardiac muscle gene expression. *Mol Cell Biol* 1992;12:1469–1479.

93. Zou Y, Chien KR. EFIA/YB-1 is a component of cardiac HF-1A binding activity and positively regulates transcription of the myosin light-chain 2v gene. *Mol Cell Biol* 1995;15:2972–2982.

94. Chen CY, Schwartz RJ. Competition between negative acting YY1 versus positive acting serum response factor and tinman homologue Nkx-2.5 regulates cardiac alpha-actin promoter activity. *Mol Endocrinol* 1997;11:812–822.

95. Lee TC, Chow K-L, Fang P, Schwartz RJ. Activation of skeletal α-actin gene transcription: the cooperative formation of serum response factor-binding complexes over positive *cis*-acting promoter serum response elements displaces a negative-acting nuclear factor enriched in replicating myoblasts and nonmyogenic cells. *Mol Cell Biol* 1991;11:5090–5100.

96. Vincent CK, Gualberto A, Patel CV, Walsh K. Different regulatory sequences control creatine kinase-M gene expression in directly injected skeletal and cardiac muscle. *Mol Cell Biol* 1993;13:1264–1272.

4. The Role of Interleukin-6 in the Failing Heart

Kai C. Wollert, MD and Helmut Drexler, MD

Department of Cardiology and Angiology, Medizinische
Hochschule Hannover, Hannover, Germany

Introduction

Traditional concepts of the pathophysiology of CHF have focussed on hemodynamic abnormalities and the activation of neurohormonal systems, such as the sympathetic nervous system the renin-angiotensin system. These concepts have provided the scientific rationale for using β-blockers and ACE inhibitors in CHF. Despite these valuable treatment strategies, however, the morbidity and mortality of patients with CHF remains high. Over the last decade it has been recognized that several cytokine systems are activated in patients with CHF. These studies gave rise to the cytokine hypothesis of CHF, which predicts that cytokine activation, in addition to neurohormonal activation, contributes to the progression of CHF. In this context, clinical studies published over the past five years, have shown that plasma concentrations of IL-6 and IL-6 related cytokines are increased in patients with CHF in relation to decreasing functional status. Moreover, plasma IL-6 was shown to provide important prognostic information. At the same time, experimental studies have indicated that IL-6 and IL-6 related cytokines play a pivotal role in the regulation of cardiac myocyte hypertrophy and apoptosis. Taken together, there is now strong evidence that IL-6 and IL-6 related cytokines are intricately involved in the pathophysiology of the failing heart.

Interleukin-6—a prominent member of a large cytokine family

Interleukin-6 was originally identified as a T cell-derived cytokine promoting the terminal maturation of activated B cells to antibody-producing cells [1,2]. Fourteen years after its initial cloning, however, IL-6 has been recognized as a multifunctional cytokine which is produced by a plethora of different cell types. Moreover, it has become apparent that IL-6 is a member of larger family of structurally-related cytokines with overlapping biological effects [3]. Besides IL-6, this cytokine family encompasses IL-11, leukemia inhibitory factor (LIF), oncostatin M (OSM), ciliary neurotrophic factor (CNTF), cardiotrophin-1 (CT-1) and novel neurotrophin-1/B cell-stimulatory factor-3 (NNT-1/BSF-3), the latest family member [4–9]. A characteristic feature of the IL-6 related cytokines is their redundancy and functional pleiotropy, i.e. the fact that different cytokines exert similar and overlapping effects on a given cell and that one cytokine can promote a wide variety of biological functions on various tissues and cells [3].

The redundancy of IL-6 related cytokines can be explained on a molecular level by the use of shared receptor subunits by different family members (Fig. 1). All IL-6 related cytokines signal through multisubunit receptor complexes that share the transmembrane glycoprotein (gp) 130. Intracellular signaling is triggered either through homodimerization of gp130 (IL-6 and IL-11 receptor systems) or heterodimerization of gp130 with a structurally related protein, the LIF receptor (LIFR) (LIF, OSM, CNTF, CT-1 and NNT-1/BSF-3 receptor systems). LIF and OSM trigger intercellular signaling through a direct interaction with the receptor components gp130 and LIFR. By contrast, IL-6, IL-11, CNTF and CT-1 cannot bind to gp130 and LIFR directly, but must first associate with cytokine-specific receptor α-subunits, the IL-6 receptor (IL-6R), IL-11R, CNTFR and CT-1R, respectively [3]. The common receptor components gp130 and LIFR are expressed in virtually every tissue and cell type, which explains the functional pleiotropy of the IL-6 related cytokines *in vitro*. Individual cytokine family members and the receptor α-subunits, however, show a more restricted tissue distribution. Considering the ubiquitous expression of gp130 and LIFR, the responsiveness of a given cell or tissue to an individual member of the IL-6 cytokine family *in vivo* will therefore depend on the presence of the corresponding receptor α-subunit. For example, expression of gp130 and the IL-6R renders a cell responsive to IL-6. Importantly, IL-6 can act on cells lacking membrane-bound IL-6R after complex formation with agonistic soluble IL-6R (sIL-6R) [10]. Soluble IL-6R is generated either by translation from an alternatively spliced mRNA [11], or is released from the cell surface by proteolytic cleavage of membrane-bound IL-6R (*shedding*) [12]. The biological activity of IL-6/sIL-6R complexes is inhibited in the presence of soluble gp130, which is generated by

Douglas L. Mann. *THE ROLE OF INFLAMMATORY MEDIATORS IN THE FAILING HEART.*
Copyright © 2001. Kluwer Academic Publishers. Boston. All rights reserved.

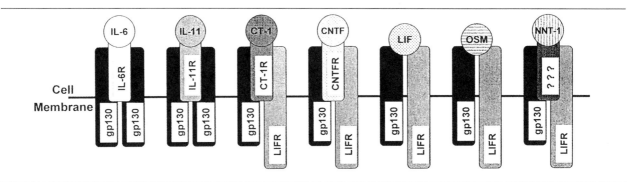

Fig. 1. IL-6 related cytokine receptor complexes. Downstream signaling is triggered by homodimerization of gp130 or heterodimerization of gp130 with the LIF receptor (LIFR). In the case of IL-6, IL-11, CNTF and CT-1, dimerization of gp130 requires a cytokine-specific receptor α-subunit.

alternative splicing and which functions as an IL-6/sIL-6R antagonist [13].

Activation of the IL-6 cytokine family in patients with heart failure

Circulating levels of IL-6 are elevated in patients with asymptomatic left ventricular dysfunction and symptomatic CHF, with a progressive increase in direct relation to decreasing functional status of the patient [14–18]. Circulating levels of soluble gp130 are increased in patients with CHF as well, and show a close relation to functional class [18]. By contrast, plasma levels of sIL-6R are similar in CHF patients and healthy control subjects [18,19]. Importantly, despite the elevated concentration of soluble gp130, which may antagonize IL-6/sIL-6R action, plasma IL-6 bioactivity is increased in patients with CHF [18]. Elevated plasma levels of IL-6 are a strong and independent prognostic marker in patients with CHF regardless of the etiology, i.e. ischemic vs. dilated cardiomyopathy [17,20]. A small study has recently shown that circulating levels of CT-1 are elevated in patients with CHF [21]. Although these results need to be confirmed in a larger cohort of patients, this study indicates that other IL-6 related cytokine(s) are induced in CHF as well. Relatively little is known regarding the cellular source and the stimuli of elevated plasma IL-6 and CT-1 levels in patients with CHF. It has been shown that plasma IL-6 concentration increases from the femoral artery to the femoral vein in patients with CHF, indicating that IL-6 is elaborated, at least in part, in the peripheral vascular bed [17]. In support of such a conclusion, it has been shown that endothelial cells and vascular smooth muscle cells are capable of producing IL-6 in vitro [22–25]. Although IL-6 related cytokines can act on target tissues in an endocrine manner, autocrine and paracrine production of these cytokines prob-

ably plays a more important role (Fig. 2). Currently, no data are available regarding the expression levels of IL-6 related cytokines and receptor systems in the failing human heart. However, studies in rats with postinfarction left ventricular dysfunction and failure indicate that IL-6 mRNA expression levels are elevated in the noninfarcted myocardium [26,27]. Similarly, cardiac CT-1 expression is increased in dogs with pacing-induced CHF [28]. These studies indicate that the failing myocardium itself may be a source of IL-6 and CT-1. In line with these observations, cardiac myocytes and fibroblasts have been shown to elaborate several IL-6 related cytokines in vitro, including IL-6, CT-1 and LIF [29–33]. Interleukin-6 related cytokines may therefore act in an autocrine and/or paracrine manner with the myocardium. Stimulation of cardiomyocytes with tumor necrosis factor (TNF)-α enhances IL-6 synthesis [34]. Considering that circulating and myocardial levels of TNF-α are increased in patients with CHF [14,35], TNF-α might be involved in the regulation of myocardial IL-6 expression. Angiotensin II enhances IL-6, CT-1 and LIF expression in cardiac myocytes and fibroblasts [30,33] and stimulates IL-6 production in vascular smooth muscle cells [24,25]. Similarly, adrenergic stimulation promotes IL-6, CT-1 and LIF synthesis in cultured cardiomyocytes [29,31]. Considering that angiotensin II and adrenergic stimulation stimulate IL-6 synthesis in vitro, and that activation of the renin-angiotensin system and the sympathetic nervous system are hallmarks of CHF [36,37], it is tempting to speculate that neurohormonal activation promotes cytokine activation in CHF. Recent studies in patients with CHF would support this concept. Plasma levels of IL-6 are positively related to circulating levels of epinephrine and norepinephrine, and negatively related to treatment with β-blockers in patients with CHF, suggesting that adrenergic

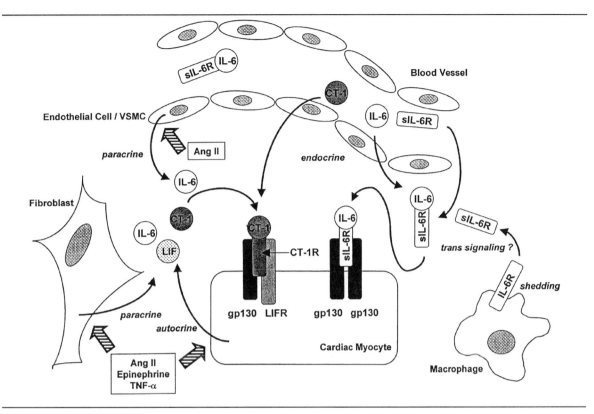

Fig. 2. *Endocrine, paracrine and autocrine action of IL-6 related cytokines. See text for details.*

activation may be linked to the induction of IL-6 [17]. Moreover, IL-6 spillover in the peripheral circulation has been shown to be independently and positively related to plasma norepinephrine concentrations, indicating that the sympathetic nervous system may stimulate IL-6 production in the periphery [17]. By contrast, myocardial expression levels of IL-6 appear to be independent from adrenergic activation, at least in rats with postinfarction CHF [27]. Treatment of patients with CHF with the angiotensin-converting enzyme inhibitor enalapril is associated with a significant decrease in IL-6 plasma levels and a modest increase in circulating levels of sIL-6R, the net effect of enalapril being a decrease in plasma IL-6 *bioactivity* [38]. Similarly, long term treatment with the angiotensin II type 1 (AT_1) receptor antagonist candesartan has been shown to reduce plasma IL-6 levels in patients with CHF [39].

While the close relation between IL-6 activation and the severity and prognosis of CHF is intriguing, IL-6 could merely represent a marker of disease severity. Experimental studies reviewed below, however, make a strong case against the notion that the activation of the IL-6 cytokine family is an epiphenomenon in CHF with little bearing on the progression of

the disease. In fact, IL-6 related cytokines have been recognized as potent inducers of cardiomyocyte hypertrophy and inhibitors of cardiomyocyte apoptosis, suggesting that IL-6 related cytokines are actively involved in the pathophysiology of CHF.

IL-6 related cytokines promote cardiac myocyte hypertrophy

It is now firmly established that IL-6 related cytokines are potent inducers of cardiac myocyte hypertrophy. The first clue linking the IL-6 cytokine family to cardiac hypertrophy was discovered by Pennica and colleagues who focussed on the isolation of novel cardiac growth factors [40]. This group had observed that medium conditioned by totipotent embryonic stem cells contained one or more substances that promoted an increase in cell size of cultured cardiomyocytes. To identify these growth promoting factors, Pennica and colleagues established a cDNA library from their embryonic cell system. The screening of a large number of cDNA clones ultimately resulted in the isolation of a novel protein that could induce cardiac myocyte hypertrophy. Accordingly, the protein was named cardiotrophin-1 [40]. Based on sequence similarity data and structural considerations, CT-1 appeared to be an IL-6 related cytokine. The subsequent identification of gp130 and LIFR as essential components of the CT-1 receptor in cardiac myocytes firmly established that CT-1 is a member of the IL-6 cytokine family [41,42].

Expression of gp130 and LIFR renders cardiomyocytes susceptible not only to CT-1 but also to other members of the IL-6 cytokine family. For example, LIF promotes a hypertrophic response in cultured cardiac myocytes that is virtually indistinguishable from the response to CT-1 [42]. Both CT-1 and LIF induce an overlapping set of immediate early genes, induce an increase in cell size and sarcomere organization and activate gene transcription and secretion of atrial natriuretic peptide (ANP). By contrast, IL-6 does not induce a hypertrophic response in cardiomyocyte culture, most likely because cardiac myocytes do not express substantial levels of the IL-6R [42,43]. However, in the presence of sIL-6R, cultured cardiac myocytes readily become responsive to IL-6 stimulation [42,44]. If these findings obtained in cultured cardiomyocytes are extrapolated to the *in vivo* situation, the susceptibility of cardiac myocytes to IL-6 mediated effects will depend on the availability of sIR-6R within the myocardium (Fig. 2). Soluble IL-6R has been detected in the plasma of patients with CHF and may permit circulating or locally produced IL-6 to act on cardiac myocytes *in vivo* [18,19]. Conceivably, sIL-6R may also be produced by neighboring cells, e.g. mononuclear cells, in a paracrine manner, and promote IL-6 action on cardiac myocytes (*trans* signaling). While such a mechanism has not been demonstrated in the failing heart, the potential importance of *trans* signaling has been established in other pathophysiological situations, e.g. in chronic inflammatory bowel disease [45].

In cardiomyocytes, like in other cell types, ligand-induced gp130 dimerization results in the activation of several intracellular signaling cascades, most notably the Janus kinase (Jak)—signal transducer and activator of transcription (STAT) pathway and the mitogen-activated protein (MAP) kinase pathways, including ERK1/2, JNK and p38 kinases [46–50] (Fig. 3). In cardiomyocytes, ligand-induced homo- or heterodimerization of gp130 induces a rapid activation and auto/transphosphorylation of the gp130-associated Janus kinases Jak1 and Jak2 [46–47]. The Jaks then phosphorylate gp130 and LIFR at cytoplasmic tyrosine residues, thereby creating docking sites for the SH2 domain containing transcription factors of the STAT family. Recruited STATs then become tyrosine phosphorylated and form homo- or heterodimers which translocate from the cytoplasm into the

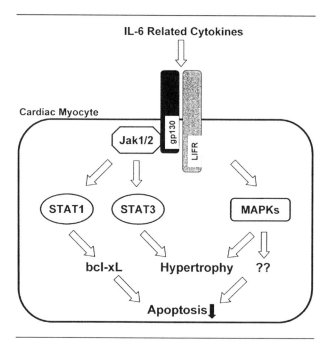

Fig. 3.   *Activation of Jak-STAT and MAPK signal transduction pathways in cardiac myocytes by IL-6 related cytokines. Induction of hypertrophy and inhibition of apoptosis are mediated by divergent signaling pathways (see text for details).*

nucleus, where they regulate target gene transcription [51]. In cardiomyocytes dimerization of gp130 and activation of Jak1/2 is quickly followed by tyrosine phosphorylation and nuclear translocation of STAT1α/β and STAT3 [46,47]. Overexpression of dominant negative STAT3 or pharmacological inhibition of MAP kinase pathways in cardiac myocytes inhibit the increase in protein synthesis and atrial natriuretic peptide expression in response to IL-6 related cytokines, suggesting that the Jak-STAT and MAP kinase signal transduction pathways are both critical for the induction of cardiac myocyte hypertrophy [49]. CT-1 has been shown to increase angiotensinogen expression via STAT3 in cardiac myocytes [52]. Interestingly, the AT_1 receptor antagonist losartan attenuated CT-1 induced cardiomyocyte hypertrophy, suggesting that autocrine production of angiotensin II might contribute to CT-1 induced cardiomyocyte hypertrophy [52].

Pan and colleagues have recently demonstrated that mechanical stretch induces a rapid phosphorylation, i.e. activation, of gp130 and STAT3 in cultured cardiomyocytes [53]. Preincubation of cardiac myocytes with a gp130 blocking antibody prevented the activation of STAT3, indicating a requirement for IL-6 related cytokines in this early response to mechanical stretch [53]. Overexpression of STAT3 has been shown to be sufficient to induce a hypertrophic response in cultured cardiac myocytes [49]. These data therefore suggest a potential role for the IL-6 cytokine family in promoting cardiomyocyte hypertrophy in response to mechanical stress. This hypothesis is further supported by the observation that mechanical stretch augments the expression of IL-6, CT-1 and LIF in cardiac myocytes [53].

Several studies indicate that IL-6 related cytokines are involved in the regulation of cardiac hypertrophy *in vivo*. In dogs with pacing-induced CHF, left ventricular expression of CT-1 is increased and closely related to left ventricular mass [28]. Similarly, cardiac CT-1 expression is increased in the early stages of left ventricular hypertrophy in genetically hypertensive rats and remains elevated after hypertrophy has been established [54]. In patients with CHF, the decrease in interventricular septum thickness during ACE-inhibitor therapy is closely related to a decrease in plasma IL-6 bioactivity, and it has therefore been speculated that a reduction of IL-6 levels may contribute to the antihypertrophic effects of ACE inhibitors [38,55].

More direct evidence that IL-6 related cytokines signaling through gp130 promote cardiac myocyte hypertrophy *in vivo* has been obtained in double-transgenic mice overexpressing IL-6 and sIL-6R [44]. The most prominent feature of the double-transgenics is a significant increase in cardiac weights with an increase in left ventricular wall thickness and cardiomyocyte size. Similar to the *in vitro* situation, transgenic mice overexpressing IL-6 alone do not display a cardiac phenotype indicating that a simultaneous overexpression of IL-6 and sIL-6R is required to induce cardiac hypertrophy *in vivo* [44]. Hirota and colleagues have recently generated mice with a cardiac myocyte-specific inactivation (*knockout*) of gp130, the shared receptor component of all IL-6 related cytokines. Cardiac-specific gp130 knockout mice survive to adulthood, develop no apparent histological abnormalities of the heart and exhibit normal cardiac function as assessed by echocardiography [56]. In control mice, pressure overload induced by transverse aortic constriction results in a rapid tyrosine phosphorylation of STAT3 in the left ventricle, a response that is not observed in cardiac-specific gp130 knockout mice [56]. Therefore, IL-6 related cytokines signaling through gp130 are required for STAT3 activation in response to pressure overload [56], a conclusion that is further supported by the study from Pan and colleagues, showing a requirement for gp130 in stretch-induced STAT3 activation in cultured cardiomyocytes [53]. Despite the loss of STAT3 activation, however, gp130-deficient hearts display a normal induction of several hypertrophy-associated genes in response to pres-

sure overload, indicating that IL-6 related cytokines are not required for the development of pressure overload hypertrophy in vivo [56]. However, the phenotype of cardiac-specific gp130 knockout animals does not rule out that IL-6 related cytokines and gp130 play a critical role in the activation of a hypertrophic response in wild type animals. These data rather suggest that gp130-dependent and gp130-independent hypertrophic pathways exist, and gp130-independent pathways can fully substitute for gp130-dependent pathways in pressure overload hypertrophy.

IL-6 related cytokines protect cardiac myocytes from apoptosis

Congestive heart failure is generally preceded by a hypertrophic response of the myocardium, that allows the heart to maintain cardiac output despite a chronic increase in hemodynamic load. However, sustained hemodynamic overloading eventually causes a transition from hypertrophy to CHF, characterized by chamber dilatation, progressive contractile dysfunction and impaired survival. The prevalence of cardiomyocyte apoptosis is increased in the failing heart but not during the initial stage of compensatory hypertrophy which suggests that cardiac myocyte dropout by apoptosis may be one mechanism contributing to the progression of cardiac hypertrophy to CHF [57–60]. Considerable research efforts have therefore focussed on the elucidation of the molecular mechanisms regulating cardiac myocyte apoptosis. In this regard, a number of studies now provide strong evidence that IL-6 related cytokines protect cardiac myocytes from apoptotic cell death. Sheng and colleagues first discovered the cytoprotective effects of IL-6 related cytokines. This group developed an assay system in which cardiomyocyte death is induced by serum deprivation [61]. As evidenced by DNA agarose gel-electrophoresis and by in situ nick end-labeling, cardiac myocyte death following serum deprivation is primarily due to apoptosis. In this assay system, IL-6 related cytokines enhance cardiac myocyte survival by blocking apoptosis [61]. In a similar study, Stephanou and colleagues have demonstrated that CT-1 protects cultured cardiac myocytes from ischemia-induced apoptosis [62]. Little is known regarding the molecular mechanisms that mediate the cytoprotective effect of IL-6 related cytokines in cardiac myocytes (Fig. 3). In this regard, IL-6 related cytokines have been shown to upregulate the anti-apoptotic regulator bcl-xL in cardiac myocytes via a STAT1 dependent transcriptional mechanism [63]. Inhibition of the MAP kinase pathway in cardiac myocytés abolishes the survival effects of the IL-6 related cytokines in serum-deprived cardiac myocytes, indicating a requirement for MAP kinases [61]. Moreover, the cytoprotective effect of CT-1 in ischemic cardiac myocytes is associated with the induction of heat shock proteins [62]. The cardiac-specific gp130 knockout mice have provided the most compelling evidence that IL-6 related cytokines are cytoprotective *in vivo*. In the setting of chronic pressure overload, these knockout mice rapidly develop cardiac dilatation associated with a dramatic increase in mortality [56]. Hearts from control mice, by contrast, display concentric hypertrophy consistent with an adaptive physiological response. As evidenced by the normal expression of embryonic genes in response to pressure overload, the rapid chamber dilatation in cardiac-specific gp130 knockout mice is not due to an inability to activate a hypertrophic response (see above). Instead, in cardiac-specific gp130 knockout mice, cardiac deterioration is associated with a significant increase in the prevalence of cardiac myocyte apoptosis [56]. It appears therefore, that gp130-dependent signaling pathways are critical for myocyte survival and the prevention of CHF in the early stages of pressure overload.

Conclusion

Congestive heart failure is associated with increased circulating levels and enhanced myocardial production of IL-6 related cytokines. Plasma IL-6 concentrations correlate with decreasing functional status in patients with CHF and provide important prognostic information. A prevailing concept of the pathophysiology of CHF predicts that the intricate balance between cardiac myocyte hypertrophy and apoptosis determines whether compensatory myocardial hypertrophy will progress to overt CHF. IL-6 related cytokines potently regulate both sides of this equilibrium by promoting cardiomyocyte hypertrophy and protecting cardiomyocytes from apoptotic cell death, strongly suggesting that this cytokine family plays a central role in the pathophysiology and progression of CHF. Future research in this important area should focus on the critical questions whether the net effect of the IL-6 cytokine family in CHF is beneficial or detrimental, and whether augmentation or inhibition of the biological effects of the IL-6 related cytokines might reduce morbidity and mortality of patients with CHF.

References

1. Hirano T, Taga T, Nakano N, Yasukawa K, Kashiwamura S, Shimizu K, Nakajima K, Pyun KH, Kishimoto T. Purification to homogeneity and charac-

terization of human B-cell differentiation factor (BCDF or BSFp-2). *Proc Natl Acad Sci USA* 1985;82:5490–5494.
2. Hirano T, Yasukawa K, Harada H, Taga T, Watanabe Y, Matsuda T, Kashiwamura S, Nakajima K, Koyama K, Iwamatsu A, Tsunasawa S, Sakiyama F, Matsui H, Takahara Y, Taniguchi T, Kishimoto T. Complementary DNA for a novel human interleukin (BSF-2) that induces B lymphocytes to produce immunoglobulin. *Nature* 1986;324:73–76.
3. Kishimoto T, Akira S. Narazaki M, Taga T. Interleukin-6 family of cytokines and gp130. *Blood* 1995;86:1243–1254.
4. Paul SR, Bennett F, Calvetti JA, Kelleher K, Wood CR, O'Hara RM, Leary AC, Sibley B, Clark SC, Williams DA, Yang YC. Molecular cloning of a cDNA encoding interleukin 11, a stromal cell-derived lymphopoietic and hematopoietic cytokine. *Proc Natl Acad Sci USA* 1990;87:7512–7516.
5. Gearing DP, Gough NM, King JA, Hilton DJ, Nicola NA, Simpson RJ, Nice EC, Kelso A, Metcalf D. Molecular cloning and expression of cDNA encoding a murine myeloid leukaemia inhibitory factor (LIF). *EMBO J* 1987;6:3995–4002.
6. Malik N, Kallestad JC, Gunderson NL, Austin SD, Neubauer MG, Ochs V, Marquardt H, Zarling JM, Shoyab M, Wei CM, Linsley PS, Rose TM. Molecular cloning, sequence analysis, and functional expression of a novel growth regulator, oncostatin M. *Mol Cell Biol* 1989;9:2847–2853.
7. Stöckli KA, Lottspeich F, Sendtner M, Masiakowski P, Carroll P, Götz R, Lindholm D, Thoenen H. Molecular cloning, expression and regional distribution of rat ciliary neurotrophic factor. *Nature* 1989;342:920–923.
8. Pennica D, King KL, Shaw KJ, Luis E, Rullamas J, Luoh SM, Darbonne WC, Knutzon DS, Yen R, Chien KR, Baker JB, Wood WI. Expression cloning of cardiotrophin 1, a cytokine that induces cardiac myocyte hypertrophy. *Proc Natl Acad Sci USA* 1995;92:1142–1146.
9. Senaldi G, Varnum BC, Sarmiento U, Starnes C, Lile J, Scully S, Guo J, Elliott G, McNinch J, Shaklee CL, Freeman D, Manu F, Simonet WS, Boone T, Chang MS. Novel neurotropin-1/B cell-stimulating factor-3. A cytokine of the IL-6 family. *Proc Natl Acad Sci USA* 1999;96:11458–11463.
10. Peters M, Jacobs S, Ehlers M, Vollmer P, Müllberg J, Wolf E, Brem G, Meyer zum Büschenfelde KH, Rose-John S. The function of the soluble interleukin 6 (IL-6) receptor *in vivo*. Sensitization of human soluble IL-6 receptor transgenic mice towards IL-6 and prolongation of the plasma half life of IL-6. *J Exp Med* 1996;183:1399–1406.
11. Müller-Newen G, Nöhne C, Keul R, Hemmann U, Müller-Esterl W, Wijdenes J, Brakenhoff JPJ, Hart MHL, Heinrich PC. Purification and characterization of the soluble interleukin-6 receptor from human plasma and identification of an isoform generated through alternative splicing. *Eur J Biochem* 1996;236:837–842.
12. Müllberg J, Durie FH, Otten-Evans C, Alderson MR, Rose-John S, Cosman D, Black RA, Mohler KM. A metalloproteinase inhibitor blocks shedding of all IL-6 receptor and the p60 TNF receptor. *J Immunol* 1995;155:5198–5205.

13. Narazaki M, Yasukawa K, Saito T, Ohsugi Y, Fukui H, Koishihara Y, Yancopoulos GD, Taga T, Kishimoto T. Soluble forms of the interleukin-6 signal-transducing receptor component gp130 in human serum possessing a potential to inhibit signals through membrane anchored gp130. *Blood* 1993;82:1120–1126.

14. Torre-Amione G, Kapadia S, Benedict C, Oral H, Young JB, Mann DL. Proinflammatory cytokine levels in patients with depressed left ventricular ejection fraction. A report from the studies of left ventricular dysfunction (SOLVD). *J Am Coll Cardiol* 1996;27:1201–1206.

15. Munger MA, Johnson B, Amber IJ, Callahan KS, Gilbert EM. Circulating concentrations of proinflammatory cytokines in mild or moderate heart failure secondary to ischemic or idiopathic dilated cardiomyopathy. *Am J Cardiol* 1996;77:723–727.

16. MacGowan GA, Mann DL, Kormos RL, Feldman AM, Murali S. Circulating interleukin-6 in severe heart failure. *Am J Cardiol* 1997;79:1128–1131.

17. Tsutamoto T, Hisanaga T, Wada A, Maeda K, Ohnishi M, Fukai D, Mabuchi N, Sawaki M, Kinoshita M. Interleukin-6 spillover in the peripheral circulation increases with the severity of heart failure, and the high plasma level of interleukin-6 is an important prognostic predictor in patients with congestive heart failure. *J Am Coll Cardiol* 1998;31:391–398.

18. Aukrust P, Ueland T, Lien E, Bendtzen K, Müller F, Andreassen AK, Nordoy I, Aass H, Espevik T, Simonsen S, Froland SS, Gullestad L. Cytokine network in congestive heart failure secondary to ischemic or idiopathic dilated cardiomyopathy. *Am J Cardiol* 1999;83:376–382.

19. Dibbs Z, Thornby J, White BG, Mann DL. Natural variability of circulating levels of cytokines and cytokine receptors in patients with heart failure. Implications for clinical trials. *J Am Coll Cardiol* 1999;33:1935–1942.

20. Orus J, Roig E, Perez-Villa F, Pare C, Azqueta M, Filella X, Heras M, Sanz G. Prognostic value of serum cytokines in patients with congestive heart failure. *J Heart Lung Transplant* 2000;19:419–425.

21. Talwar S, Downie PF, Squire IB, Barnett DB, Davies JD, Ng LL. An immunoluminometric assay for cardiotrophin-1. A newly identified cytokine is present in normal human plasma and is increased in heart failure. *Biochem Biophys Res Comm* 1999;261:567–571.

22. Jirik FR, Podor TJ, Hirano T. Bacterial lipopolysaccharide and inflammatory mediators augment IL-6 secretion by human endothelial cells. *J Immunol* 1989;142:144–147.

23. Xin X, Cai Y, Matsumoto K, Agui T. Endothelin-induced interleukin-6 production by rat aortic endothelial cells. *Endocrinology* 1995;136:132–137.

24. Han Y, Runge MS, Brasier AR. Angiotensin II induces interleukin-6 transcription in vascular smooth muscle cells through pleiotropic activation of nuclear factor-κB transcription factors. *Circ Res* 1999;84:695–703.

25. Schieffer B, Schieffer E, Hilfiker-Kleiner D, Hilfiker A, Kovanen PT, Kaartinen M, Nussberger J, Harringer W, Drexler H. Expression of angiotensin II and interleukin 6 in human coronary atherosclerotic plaques. Potential implications for inflammation and plaque instability. *Circulation* 2000;101:1372–1378.

26. Ono K, Matsumori A, Shioi T, Furukawa Y, Sasayama S. Cytokine gene expression after myocardial infarction in rat hearts. Possible implication in left ventricular remodeling. *Circulation* 1998;98:149–156.

27. Prabhu SD, Chandrasekar B, Murray DR, Freeman GL. β-Adrenergic blockade in developing heart failure. Effects of myocardial inflammatory cytokines, nitric oxide, and remodeling. *Circulation* 2000;101:2103–2109.

28. Jougasaki M, Tachibana I, Luchner A, Leskinen H, Redfield MM, Burnett JC. Augmented cardiotrophin-1 in experimental congestive heart failure. *Circulation* 2000;101:14–17.

29. Yamauchi-Takihara K, Ihara Y, Ogata A, Yoshizaki K, Azuma J, Kishimoto T. Hypoxic stress induces cardiac myocyte-derived interleukin-6. *Circulation* 1995;91:1520–1524.

30. Sano M, Fukuda K, Kodama H, Takahashi T, Kato T, Hakuno D, Sato T, Manabe T, Tahara S, Ogawa S. Autocrine/paracrine secretion of IL-6 family cytokines causes angiotensin II-induced delayed STAT3 activation. *Biochem Biophys Res Comm* 2000;269:798–802.

31. Funamoto M, Hishinuma S, Fujio Y, Matsuda Y, Kunisada K, Oh H, Negoro S, Tone E, Kishimoto T, Yamauchi-Takihara K. Isolation and characterization of the murine cardiotrophin-1 gene. Expression and norepinephrine-induced transcriptional activation. *J Mol Cell Cardiol* 2000;32:1275–1284.

32. Kuwahara K, Saito Y, Harada M, Ishikawa M, Ogawa E, Miyamoto Y, Hamanaka I, Kamitani S, Kajiyama N, Takahashi N, Nakagawa O, Masuda I, Nakao K. Involvement of cardiotrophin-1 in cardiac myocyte-nonmyocyte interactions during hypertrophy of rat cardiac myocytes *in vitro*. *Circulation* 1999;100:1116–1124.

33. Sano M, Fukuda K, Kodama H, Pan J, Saito M, Matsuzaki J, Takahashi T, Makino S, Kato T, Ogawa S. Interleukin-6 family of cytokines mediate angiotensin II-induced cardiac hypertrophy in rodent cardiomyocytes. *J Biol Chem* 2000;275:29717–29723.

34. Gwechenberger M, Mendoza LH, Youker KA, Frangogiannis NG, Smith CW, Michael LH, Entman ML. Cardiac myocytes produce interleukin-6 in culture and in viable border of reperfused infarctions. *Circulation* 1999;99:546–551.

35. Torre-Amione G, Kapadia S, Lee J, Durand JB, Bies RD, Young JB, Mann DL. Tumor necrosis factor-α and tumor necrosis factor receptors in the failing human heart. *Circulation* 1996;93:704–711.

36. Wollert K, Drexler H. The renin-angiotensin system and experimental heart failure. *Cardiovasc Res* 1999;43:838–849.

37. Bristow MR. β-Adrenergic receptor blockade in chronic heart failure. *Circulation* 2000;101:558–569.

38. Gullestad L, Aukrust P, Ueland T, Espevik T, Yee G, Vagelos R, Froland SS, Fowler M. Effect of high- versus low-dose angiotensin converting enzyme inhibition on cytokine levels in chronic heart failure. *J Am Coll Cardiol* 1999;34:2061–2067.

39. Tsutamoto T, Wada A, Maeda K, Mabuchi N, Hayashi M, Tsutsui T, Ohnishi M, Sawaki M,

Fujii M, Matsumoto T, Kinoshita M. Angiotensin II type 1 receptor antagonist decreases plasma levels of tumor necrosis factor alpha, interleukin-6 and soluble adhesion molecules in patients with chronic heart failure. *J Am Coll Cardiol* 2000;35:714–721.

40. Pennica D, King KL, Shaw KJ, Luis E, Rullamas J, Luoh SM, Darbonne WC, Knutzon DS, Yen R, Chien KR, Baker JB, Wood WI. Expression cloning of cardiotrophin 1, a cytokine that induces cardiac myocyte hypertrophy. *Proc Natl Acad Sci USA* 1995;92:1142–1146.

41. Pennica D, Shaw KJ, Swanson TA, Moore MW, Shelton DL, Zioncheck KA, Rosenthal A, Taga T, Paoni NF, Wood WI. Cardiotrophin-1. Biological activities and binding to the leukemia inhibitory factor receptor/gp130 signaling complex. *J Biol Chem* 1995;270:10915–10922.

42. Wollert KC, Taga T, Saito M, Narazaki M, Kishimoto T, Glembotski CC, Vernallis AB, Health JK, Pennica D, Wood WI, Chien KR. Cardiotrophin-1 activates a distinct form of cardiac muscle cell hypertrophy. Assembly of sarcomeric units in series via gp130/leukemia inhibitory factor receptor-dependent pathways. *J Biol Chem* 1996;271:9535–9545.

43. Saito M, Yoshida K, Hibi M, Taga T, Kishimoto T. Molecular cloning of a murine IL-6 receptor-associated signal transducer, gp130, and its regulated expression *in vivo*. *J Immunol* 1992;148:4066–4071.

44. Hirota H, Yoshida K, Kishimoto T, Taga T. Continuous activation of gp130, a signal-transducing receptor component for interleukin 6-related cytokines, causes myocardial hypertrophy in mice. *Proc Natl Acad Sci USA* 1995;92:4862–4866.

45. Atreya R, Mudter J, Finotto S, Müllberg J, Jostock T, Wirtz S, Schütz M, Bartsch B, Holtmann M, Becker C, Strand D, Czaja J, Schlaak JF, Lehr HA, Autschbach F, Schürmann G, Nishimoto N, Yoshizaki K, Ito H, Kishimoto T, Galle PR, Rose-John S, Neurath MF. Blockade of interleukin 6 trans signaling suppresses T-cell resistance against apoptosis in chronic intestinal inflammation. Evidence in Crohn disease and experimental colitis *in vivo*. *Nature Med* 2000;6:583–588.

46. Kunisada K, Hirota H, Fujio Y, Matsui H, Tani Y, Yamauchi-Takihara K, Kishimoto T. Activation of JAK-STAT and MAP kinases by leukemia inhibitory factor through gp130 in cardiac myocytes. *Circulation* 1996;94:2626–2632.

47. Kodama H, Fukuda K, Pan J, Makino S, Baba A, Hori S, Ogawa S. Leukemia inhibitory factor, a potent cardiac hypertrophic cytokine, activates the JAK/STAT pathway in rat cardiomyocytes. *Circ Res* 1997;81:656–663.

48. Wollert KC, Chien KR. Cardiotrophin-1 and the role of gp130-dependent signaling pathways in cardiac growth and development. *J Mol Med* 1997;75:492–501.

49. Kunisada K, Tone E, Fujio Y, Matsui H, Yamauchi-Takihara K, Kishimoto T. Activation of gp130 transduces hypertrophic signals via STAT3 in cardiac myocytes. *Circulation* 1998;98:346–352.

50. Nemoto S, Sheng Z, Lin A. Opposing effects of Jun Kinase and p38 mitogen-activated protein kinases

on cardiomyocyte hypertrophy. *Mol Cell Biol* 1998;18:3518–3526.

51. Heinrich PC, Behrmann I, Müller-Newen G, Schaper F, Graeve L. Interleukin-6-type cytokine signalling through the gp130/Jak/STAT pathway. *Biochem J* 1998;334:297–314.

52. Fukuzawa J, Booz GW, Hunt RA, Shimizu N, Karoor V, Baker KM, Dostal DE. Cardiotrophin-1 increases angiotensinogen mRNA in rat cardiac myocytes through STAT3. An autocrine loop for hypertrophy. *Hypertension* 2000;35:1191–1196.

53. Pan J, Fukuda K, Saito M, Matsuzaki J, Kodama H, Sano M, Takahashi T, Kato T, Ogawa S. Mechanical stretch activates the JAK/STAT pathway in rat cardiomyocytes. *Circ Res* 1999;84:1127–1136.

54. Ishikawa M, Saito Y, Miyamoto Y, Harada M, Kuwahara K, Ogawa E, Nakagawa O, Hamanaka I, Kajiyama N, Takahashi N, Masuda I, Hashimoto T, Sakai O, Hosoya T, Nakao K. A heart-specific increase in cardiotrophin-1 gene expression precedes the establishment of ventricular hypertrophy in genetically hypertensive rats. *J Hypertens* 1999; 17:807–816.

55. Young JB. Angiotensin-converting enzyme inhibitors and cytokines in heart failure. Dose and effect? *J Am Coll Cardiol* 1999;34:2068–2071.

56. Hirota H, Chen J, Betz UAK, Rajewsky K, Gu Y, Ross J, Müller W, Chien KR. Loss of a gp130 cardiac muscle cell survival pathway is a critical event in the onset of heart failure during biomechanical stress. *Cell* 1999;97:189–198.

57. Cheng W, Kajstura J, Nitahara JA, Li B, Reiss K, Liu Y, Clark WA, Krajewski S, Reed JC, Olivetti G, Anversa P. Programmed myocyte cell death affects the viable myocardium after infarction in rats. *Exp Cell Res* 1996;226:316–327.

58. Li Z, Bing OHL, Long X, Robinson KG, Lakatta EG. Increased cardiomyocyte apoptosis during the transition to heart failure in the spontaneously hypertensive rat. *Am J Physiol* 1997;272:H2313–H2319.

59. Olivetti G, Abbi R, Quaini F, Kajstura J, Cheng W, Nitahara JA, Quaini E, di Loreto C, Beltrami CA, Krajewski S, Reed JC, Anversa P. Apoptosis in the failing human heart. *N Engl J Med* 1997;336:1131–1141.

60. Williams RS. Apoptosis and heart failure. *N Engl J Med* 1999;341:759–760.

61. Sheng Z, Knowlton K, Chen J, Hoshijima M, Brown JH, Chien KR. Cardiotrophin-1 inhibition of cardiac myocyte apoptosis via a mitogen-activated protein kinase-dependent pathway. Divergence from downstream CT-1 signals for myocardial cell hypertrophy. *J Biol Chem* 1997;272:5783–5791.

62. Stephanou A, Brar B, Heads R, Knight RD, Marber MS, Pennica D, Latchman DS. Cardiotrophin-1 induces heat shock protein accumulation in cultured cardiac myocytes and protects them from stressful stimuli. *J Mol Cell Cardiol* 1998;30:849–855.

63. Fujio Y, Kunisada K, Hirota H, Yamauchi-Takihara K, Kishimoto T. Signals through gp130 upregulate bcl-x gene expression via STAT1-binding cis-element in cardiac myocytes. *J Clin Invest* 1997;99:2898–2905.

5. The Role of Nitric Oxide in the Failing Heart

Walter J. Paulus, MD, PhD, FESC

Cardiovascular Center, O.L.V. Ziekenhuis, Aalst, Belgium

Introduction: myocardial contractile effects of nitric oxide

Most experimental studies looking at contractile effects of nitric oxide (NO) tried to label NO as a positive or a negative inotrope for myocardial contractile performance [1]. In contrast to the well-defined vasodilator action of NO in the vasculature, experimental studies on the myocardial contractile effects of NO yielded contradictory results reporting both positive and negative inotropic actions [2]. This variability of the myocardial contractile response to NO resulted from methodological differences such as the source of NO, the amount of NO to which the experimental preparation was exposed, the presence of simultaneous neurohormonal stimuli and the prevailing redox balance. Although the initial *in vitro* experiments mainly suggested a negative inotropic effect of NO [3], studies looking at left ventricular (LV) contractile performance in humans never observed a change in a LV contractility index such as $LVdP/dt_{max}$ during intracoronary infusion of NO-donors [4,5], of inhibitors of NO synthase (NOS) [6] or of substance P [7], which triggers endothelial NO release. Only following pretreatment with β-agonists but not under baseline conditions did intracoronary infusion of substance P [8] or of a NOS inhibitor [9,10] result in significant changes in $LVdP/dt_{max}$ consistent with a negative inotropic effect of NO.

Conclusions on *in vitro* myocardial contractile effects of NO were frequently based on an incomplete analysis of myocardial performance looking only at the extent of shortening of unloaded isolated cardiomyocytes without considering effects of NO on isometric tension development or on the relaxation phase of myocardial contraction. In fact, the original observations on the contractile effects of NO in an isolated cardiac muscle strip preparation that allowed for variable contraction modes (both isotonic and isometric) and for analysis of the time course of the contraction-relaxation sequence, revealed a very unique way in which NO affected cardiac muscle performance [11]. *NO had no effect on the rate of rise of isometric tension (dT/dt_{max}) but reduced peak isometric tension because of earlier onset of isometric tension decay* (Fig. 1). NO therefore modified myocardial contractile performance through a unique relaxation-hastening effect. Only natriuretic peptides [12], which like NO raise myocardial cGMP, or a decrease in muscle preload induced a similar relaxation-hastening effect without change in dT/dt_{max}. A relaxation-hastening effect was also observed in the human heart during intracoronary infusions of NO-donor substances [4,5] or of substance P [7]. This relaxation-hastening effect abbreviated LV contraction, reduced the magnitude of the late-systolic LV pressure-wave and caused a $\pm 10\,mmHg$ fall in LV end-systolic pressure (Fig. 1). This fall in LV end-systolic pressure induced a downward and rightward shift of the LV end-systolic pressure–volume relation [7]. Although this rightward shift of the LV end-systolic pressure–volume relation was theoretically consistent with a negative inotropic effect, it was probably beneficial for the ejecting left ventricle because it reduced the mechanical work wasted in contracting against reflected arterial pressure waves. Pretreatment with β-agonists increased the NO-induced LV relaxation hastening effect and the fall in LV end-systolic pressure ($\pm 20\,mmHg$) [8].

In humans, the LV relaxation-hastening effect of NO was accompanied by an effect of NO on diastolic LV distensibility. During intracoronary infusions of NO-donors or of substance P [4,5,7] the LV diastolic pressure–volume relation shifted rightward consistent with increased LV diastolic distensibility. Direct effects of NO on diastolic myocardial distensibility were also observed in isolated rat or rabbit cardiomyocytes, in intact guinea pig, rat or rabbit hearts and in anaesthetized dogs. In isolated rat cardiomyocytes, a reduction in diastolic tone was observed following exposure to sodium nitroprusside [13] and following exposure to 8 bromo-cyclicGMP, the second messenger of NO [14]. In isolated rabbit cardiomyocytes, exposure to lipopolysaccharides [15] or to natriuretic peptides [16] resulted in altered cell volume through a NO and cyclicGMP-mediated mechanism. These alterations in cell volume were associated with increased LV diastolic distensibility. In isolated guinea pig hearts, LV volume loading induced a rise in NO concentration of the coronary effluent [17] and addition of a specific inhibitor of NOS to the coronary perfusate caused an elevation of LV end-diastolic pressure and a reduction in LV preload reserve [18]. The rise in NO concentration of the coronary effluent during LV volume loading was consistent with the increased diastolic intramyocardial NO concentrations measured by a porphyrinic sensor

Douglas L. Mann. *THE ROLE OF INFLAMMATORY MEDIATORS IN THE FAILING HEART.*
Copyright © 2001. Kluwer Academic Publishers. Boston. All rights reserved.

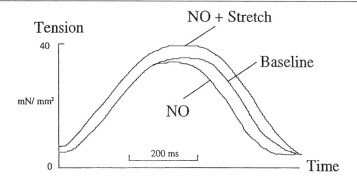

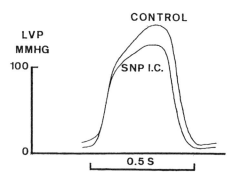

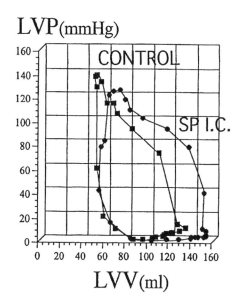

Fig. 1.   Top panel: Effects of NO on isolated papillary muscle isometric contraction. NO has no effect on the rate of rise of isometric tension but causes earlier onset of isometric tension decay with concomitant reduction in peak isometric tension. These effects of NO are counteracted by an increase in muscle preload (NO + Stretch). Middle panel: Effects of an intracoronary (I.C.) infusion of SNP (Sodium Nitroprusside) on LV pressure. There is no effect of NO on the rate of rise of LV pressure but an earlier onset of isovolumic LV pressure decay with reduction of peak and end-systolic LV pressures unrelated to systemic vasodilation. Lower panel: Effects on the LV pressure (LVP)-volume (LVV) relation of endothelially released NO during intracoronary (I.C.) infusion of substance P (SP). During I.C. infusion of SP, there is a small right and downward displacement of the end-systolic pressure–volume point and a right and downward displacement of the diastolic pressure–volume relation consistent with an increase in diastolic LV distensibility.

in the wall of the beating rabbit heart following release of a vena cava occluder [19]. In anaesthetized dogs, NOS inhibition increased diastolic LV stiffness and L-arginine resulted in opposite effects [17]. Changes in diastolic LV distensibility have been observed not only following acute administration of a NOS inhibitor but also following chronic NOS blockade. In rats receiving eight weeks of treatment with a NOS inhibitor, the diastolic LV pressure volume relation shifted upward with a significant reduction in LV unstressed volume and no increase in LV mass despite the elevated blood pressure [20].

Based on the foregoing experimental and clinical evidence, contractile effects of NO relevant to the failing human heart consist of:

1) a LV relaxation-hastening effect, which abbreviates LV contraction and slightly reduces LV end-systolic pressure thereby preventing wastage of LV mechanical work against reflected late-systolic arterial pressure waves;
2) a LV cardiodepressant effect (fall in $LVdP/dt_{max}$ and rightward shift of the LV end-systolic pressure–volume relation) only following pretreatment with β-adrenergic agonists but not under baseline conditions;
3) a LV distensibility-increasing effect, which augments the LV Frank-Starling response or LV preload reserve.

Myocardial effects of nitric oxide in experimental and clinical heart failure

Contractile effects. In patients with dilated nonischemic cardiomyopathy [21], an intracoronary infusion of substance P, which releases NO from the coronary endothelium, caused no change in $LVdP/dt_{max}$ but induced an acute rightward displacement of the LV diastolic pressure–volume relation. In patients with elevated baseline LV filling pressures, this rightward displacement of the LV diastolic pressure–volume relation increased LV stroke volume and LV stroke work consistent with augmentation of LV preload reserve [21]. Intracoronary infusion of a NOS inhibitor in patients with dilated cardiomyopathy [6] resulted in a rise in $LVdP/dt_{max}$ only following pretreatment with β-agonists but not under baseline conditions. The absence of an effect on baseline $LVdP/dt_{max}$ in both studies suggests the myocardial effects of elevated plasma catecholamines in heart failure to be offset by a simultaneous reduction in myocardial $\beta1$-receptors and/or a simultaneous increase in myocardial G_i-proteins. In a dog model of pacing-induced heart failure, cardiac NO production fell after 4 weeks of pacing and this fall was accompanied by a significant rise in LV end-diastolic pressure and a fall in LV stroke work again consistent with NO-related effects on LV diastolic distensibility and preload reserve [22].

Energetic effects. Altered energetics of the failing heart are characterized by: 1) a reduction in creatine kinase activity, phosphocreatine levels and total creatine levels; 2) an alteration in mitochondrial function; 3) a switch in myocardial substrate utilisation from free fatty acids to glucose. NO has recently been shown to interfere with all three derangements of energetics of failing myocardium. In isolated rat hearts, perfusion with a NO donor resulted in inhibition of creatine kinase activity and a decrease in contractile performance during inotropic stimulation [23]. A reduction of creatine kinase activity raised free intramyocardial ADP, which correlated closely with LV end-diastolic pressure [24]. In conscious dogs, NO synthase inhibitors increased myocardial oxygen consumption [25] probably because of reduced inhibition of cytochrome C oxidase, the terminal enzyme of the mitochondrial respiratory chain. The lower cardiac NO production observed in advanced experimental pacing-induced heart failure therefore explained the loss of control of myocardial mitochondrial respiration [22]. In failing human myocardium, a similar modulation of oxygen consumption by endogenous NO was observed. This modulation of myocardial oxygen consumption was importantly altered by pharmacological inhibition of kinin degradation with ACE inhibitor, amlodipine or neutral endopeptidase inhibitor [26]. Proinflammatory cytokines, whose levels are frequently elevated in heart failure, have both NO-mediated and direct effects on myocardial mitochondrial function. Interleukin-1 stimulated NO production, which inhibited the mitochondrial respiratory chain in rat cardiomyocytes [27]. TNF-α activated sfingomyelinase and caused production of ceramide [28], which also inhibited the mitochondrial respiratory chain [29] and which caused cytosolic release from the mitochondria of cytochrome C, a potent inductor of apoptosis. In conscious dogs with pacing-induced heart failure, a drop in cardiac NO production was observed at the time of transition into decompensated heart failure [22]. This drop in cardiac NO production was accompanied by a switch in myocardial substrate utilisation from free fatty acids to glucose. A similar switch was also demonstrated in transgenic mice with defects in the expression of NO synthase [30].

Apoptosis and expression of fetal gene programme

In patients with ischemic or dilated cardiomyopathy, activation of myocardial apoptosis is increased [31,32]. The extent of this activation is the subject of considerable controversy [33]. NO was reported to have both proapoptotic and antiapoptotic actions on the myocardium [34]. In NOS2 knockout mice, acute cardiac rejection was attenuated and correlated with reduced apoptotic cell death [35]. In cultured cardiomyocytes, interleukin-1β and interferon-γ increased apoptosis through generation of peroxynitrite ($ONOO^-$) from NO and superoxide (O_2^-) [36,37]. $ONOO^-$ also decreased contractile performance of these cultured cardiomyocytes. The absence of a cardiodepressant effect of NO on baseline LV function in the human heart suggests an important *in vivo* protective effect of superoxide dismutase or of glutathion against $ONOO^-$ production [38] or against $ONOO^-$ toxicity because of formation of nitrosothiols [39]. Nitrosothiols are antiapoptotic because of S-nitrosation of caspases. This antiapoptotic action of NO could be of relevance to human heart failure because serum from patients with heart failure was recently demonstrated to downregulate NOS2 expression and to upregulate apoptosis in human endothelial cells [40].

In isolated cardiomyocytes, norepinephrine-induced expression of the fetal gene programme was blocked by NO, atrial natriuretic peptide and cGMP [41]. Expression of the fetal gene programme was especially deleterious for myocardial calcium handling because of deficient expression of sarcoplasmic reticular Ca^{2+} ATPase [42]. Although this effect of NO on expression of the fetal gene programme was explained by a reduction of the norepinephrine-induced calcium influx, recent evidence also suggested direct effect of NO on gene expression [43].

Altered endomyocardial nitric oxide synthase in failing myocardium

All three isoforms of NO Synthase (NOS) are expressed in failing myocardium:

Neuronal NOS (nNOS, NOS1) is mainly expressed in neural tissue and in skeletal muscle but has recently also been reported in myocardial tissue. It binds to the cytoskeletal Z-line dystrophin-sarcoglycan complex. Because of dystrophin deficiency, myocardial expression of nNOS was reduced in X-linked dilated cardiomyopathy of Duchenne's muscular dystrophy [44]. This myocardial downregulation of nNOS was accompanied by an upregulation of another isoform, namely inducible NOS (iNOS, NOS2). Dystro-

phin deficiency and cytoskeletal disruption were recently also postulated to occur in acquired cardiomyopathies following myocarditis because of specific dystrophin cleavage by enteroviral protease [45]. The reported downregulation of nNOS and upregulation of iNOS in the presence of low dystrophin could therefore also apply to other forms of dilated cardiomyopathy.

Endothelial or constitutive NOS (eNOS, cNOS, ecNOS, NOS3) is a calcium sensitive isoform present mainly in endothelial cells but also in the myocardium [46]. Experimental evidence on endomyocardial NOS3 expression and activity in heart failure provides support for the intensity of NOS3 gene expression to vary with the severity of LV dysfunction. In a pacing-induced heart failure dog model, NOS3 activity was increased after two weeks of pacing as evident from enhanced endothelium-dependent relaxations of isolated coronary artery rings [47]. In the same pacing-induced heart failure dog model, cardiac NO production was however reduced after four weeks of pacing [22]. In a postinfarction rat-failure model, cardiac NOS3 was decreased and restored to baseline level following addition of captopril to the drinking water [48]. Reduced cardiac NOS3 activity and improvement during ACE inhibitor therapy was also deduced from clinical studies on heart failure patients, which reported a decrease in the endothelium-dependent vasodilation of the coronary microvasculature [49] and an improvement of the vasodilator response during chronic quinapril therapy [50]. Direct measurements of endomyocardial NOS3 gene expression in patients with dilated cardiomyopathy yielded however conflicting results in so far that both low [51] and high [52,53] intensities of NOS3 gene expression had been reported. The divergent results of these clinical studies probably arose from different sites and modes of myocardial tissue procurement and from the varying severity of cardiomyopathic dysfunction. The site and mode of myocardial tissue procurement indeed included right ventricular tissue obtained by transvascular biopsy, right ventricular tissue excised during cardiopulmonary bypass, LV tissue obtained by transvascular biopsy and LV tissue from explanted hearts at the time of cardiac transplantation. Detection of an upregulation of myocardial NOS3, as a result of a mechanical stress applied to the left ventricle, requires LV and not right ventricular tissue as illustrated in spontaneously hypertensive rats, where NOS3 activity was upregulated in LV but not in right ventricular tissue [54]. A recent study using LV endomyocardial biopsies and studying not only end-stage heart failure patients but also patients with moderate compensated heart failure, found the intensity of NOS3 gene expression to be inversely correlated with the severity of LV dysfunction [21]. In this study, higher LV stroke volume and stroke work were observed in patients with higher LV endomyocardial NOS3 gene expression (Fig. 2). In this and one other study [52], patients on β-blocker ther-

apy also had higher NOS3 gene expression. Up-regulation of NOS3 gene expression during β-blocker therapy probably resulted from increased transcription and subcellular targeting to plasmalemmal caveolae of NOS3 as a result of reduced myocardial cAMP content [55,56].

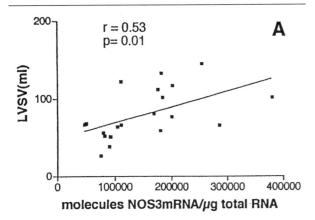

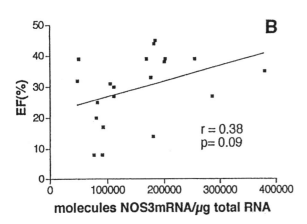

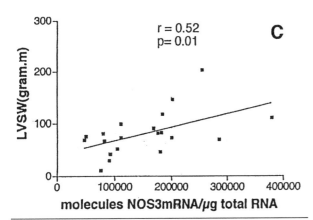

Fig. 2. Linear correlations between LV stroke volume (LVSV) (A), LV ejection fraction (EF) (B) and LV stroke work (LVSW) (C) and intensity of NOS3 mRNA expression. Reproduced with permission from ref 21.

Inducible NOS (iNOS, NOS2). Since the original demonstration of NOS2 expression in cardiomyocytes stimulated with endotoxin [57] or cytokines [58], myocardial expression of NOS2 was frequently cited as a mechanism underlying cardiodepression observed in immune-mediated conditions, despite subsequent reports, which failed to demonstrate NO-mediated negative inotropic effects following exposure to cytokines [59]. Moreover, most of the evidence for NOS2-mediated cardiodepression in immune-mediated conditions was based on experiments performed in isolated cardiomyocytes with limited anti-oxidant capacity and data demonstrating NOS2-induced cardiodepression in intact animal models or in man are either controversial or absent.

In rat or mice myocarditis models both deleterious and beneficial effects of NOS2 expression have been reported. In myosin-immunised rats, the selective NOS2-inhibitor aminoguanidine exerted a favorable hemodynamic effect, which was thought to result from avoidance of NO-related negative inotropic effects or of ONOO$^-$ production [60]. Administration of a NOS-inhibitor also resulted in reduced myocardial destruction in a murine myocarditis model [61] but NOS2 "knockout" mice had higher mortality following myocarditis [62]. This beneficial effect of NOS2 in the "knockout" mice was mainly attributed to maintenance of an appropriate inflammatory response. Immune-associated myocardial contractile depression was also investigated in conscious dogs [63,64]. Following administration of tumor necrosis factor-α, a delayed left ventricular contractile depression was observed. This contractile depression could have been consistent with cytokine-induced NOS2 expression and subsequent NO generation but actual proof using NOS inhibitors was lacking. In dogs with pacing-induced heart failure, myocardial NOS activity was significantly increased compared with control dogs. In this experimental model, administration of a NOS inhibitor had no effect on basal myocardial contractility and only augmented the inotropic response to β-adrenergic stimulation [65].

Expression of NOS2 was first reported in ventricular myocardium of patients with dilated cardiomyopathy after myocarditis [66], in allograft recipients at the time of surveillance endomyocardial biopsy [67] and subsequently in myocardium of failing hearts regardless of the underlying cause [68]. In allograft recipients undergoing surveillance endomyocardial biopsy, a Dopplerechocardiographic study [67] showed NOS2 gene expression to correlate with LV dysfunction but an invasive assessment of LV performance [69] failed to demonstrate effects of high myocardial NOS2 expression on LV ejection fraction or on LV dP/dt_{max}. In heart failure patients, NOS2 gene expression was more frequent in NYHA class II patients than in class IV patients [68] but in a subsequent study [70] high NOS2 gene expression was associated not with functional class but with low LV ejection fraction. A recent study in patients with dilated cardiomyopathy used LV endomyocardial biopsies and correlated intensity of LV endomyocardial NOS2 gene expression with LV performance [21]. The use of LV endomyocardial biopsies instead of tissue from explanted hearts allowed patients with moderate LV dysfunction also to be included in the study. This study observed a linear correlation between intensity of LV endomyocardial NOS2 gene expression and LV ejection fraction, LV stroke volume or LV stroke work (Fig. 3).

Nitric oxide synthase and the progression of left ventricular dysfunction

The parallel reduction of NOS2 and NOS3 gene expression during the progression from moderate to severe LV dysfunction [21] (Figs. 2–3) is noteworthy because in cardiomyocytes, regulators of gene expression of NOS isoenzymes usually produce opposite effects on NOS2 and NOS3 mRNA. Cytokines increase NOS2 mRNA and interferon-γ and interleukin-1β decrease NOS3 mRNA. Cyclic AMP stimulates NOS2 mRNA stability [71] and downregulates NOS3 transcription [55]. Transforming growth factor β, which is abundantly expressed in dilated cardiomyopathy, reduces NOS2 mRNA stability [72] and upregulates NOS3 mRNA stability [73]. Cytokines, neurohormones and growth factors are therefore probably not involved in the observed parallel downregulation of gene expression of NOS isoenzymes in patients with severe left ventricular dysfunction.

Downregulation of myocardial gene expression in severe LV dysfunction has also been reported for other genes. Lower levels of protooncogenes were observed in peroperative biopsy samples of patients with aortic regurgitation and major LV dysfunction [74] and a fall in expression of gp130 and of interleukin-6 related cardiotrophin-1 accompanies transition to a maladaptive response in LV hemodynamic overload [75].

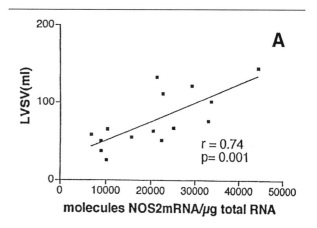

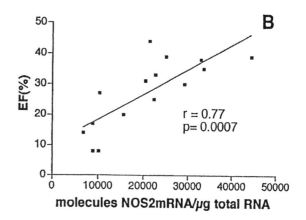

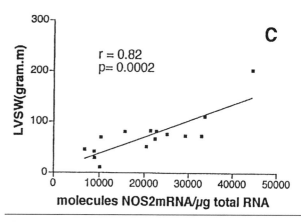

Fig. 3. *Linear correlations between LV stroke volume (LVSV) (A), LV ejection fraction (EF) (B) and LV stroke work (LVSW) (C) and intensity of NOS2 mRNA expression in patients with dilated cardiomyopathy and elevated (>16 mmHg) LV end-diastolic pressure. Reproduced with permission from ref 21.*

Downregulation of gene expression in advanced LV dysfunction could result from reduction of the cardiomyocyte population because of apoptotic cell death or from altered transmission of wall stress from the extracellular matrix to the cardiomyocytes. The remodeling process of progressive LV cardiomyopathic dysfunction involves increased extracellular matrix degradation and turnover because of upregulation of certain matrix metalloproteinases and downregulation of tissue inhibitors of metalloproteinases [76]. This leads to disruption of the collagen weave around individual myocytes [77] and to malalignment or slippage of myocytes. Disruption of the collagen weave could alter transmission of LV wall stress to the cardiomyocytes and disturb wall stress-induced gene expression because of an altered cascade of signals originating from the collagen fibers and descending to sarcolemmal integrins, to cytoskeletal proteins and to nuclear membranes [78].

Nitric oxide synthase and LV preload reserve

In patients with dilated nonischaemic cardiomyopathy, linear correlations were observed between left ventricular stroke volume or stroke work and intensity of endomyocardial NOS2 or NOS3 gene expression [21] (Figs. 2 and 3) especially if the hearts were operating at elevated LV filling pressures. These correlations between myocardial NOS gene expression and LV stroke volume or stroke work resulted from a direct myocardial action of NO because in these patients an intracoronary infusion of substance P, which releases NO from the coronary endothelium, induced an acute rightward displacement of the LV end-diastolic pressure–volume relation and a concomitant increase in LV stroke volume and LV stroke work [21].

Patients with dilated cardiomyopathy are highly dependent on preload recrutable LV stroke work to compensate for reduced inotropic reserve [79]. This enhancement of preload recrutable LV stroke work results from a rightward displacement of the diastolic LV pressure–volume relation [80]. Limitation of this rightward displacement leads to development of a restrictive LV filling pattern, which is accompanied by exacerbation of symptoms and poor prognosis [81,82]. Because of NO's ability to shift the diastolic LV pressure–volume relationship rightward, a reduced intensity of LV endomyocardial NOS gene expression could underlie the development of a restrictive LV filling pattern in patients with dilated cardiomyopathy. In these patients, LV endomyocardial NOS2 gene expression indeed appeared to be inversely related to left ventricular diastolic stiffness ($p = 0.003$; $r = 0.50$) [83]. In this correlation, data scatter arose from low NOS2 gene expression observed in some patients with low LV diastolic stiffness. These patients were all

operating at low LV end-diastolic wall stress (EDWS). Figure 4 plots NOS2 gene expression in function of LVEDWS for different levels of LV diastolic stiffness. In Figure 4, patients with high LV diastolic stiffness (Stiffness-Modulus $> 300 \, kdyne/cm^2$) clustered in the upper left hand corner of the graph, patients with intermediate values occupied the middle portion of the graph and patients with low LV diastolic stiffness (Stiffness-Modulus $< 150 \, kdyne/cm^2$) clustered in the lower right hand corner of the graph. Because of this clustering in accordance to LV diastolic stiffness, the slope of the NOS2 gene expression-LVEDWS relation appeared to correlate more closely with LV diastolic stiffness ($p < 0.0001$; $r = 0.80$) than NOS2 gene expression itself.

Higher LV diastolic stiffness because of lower endomyocardial NOS gene expression explains the worsening of the hemodynamic phenotype in patients with dilated cardiomyopathy. High expression of endomyocardial NOS could indeed have resulted in a substantial NO-induced rightward displacement of the diastolic LV pressure–volume relation, which kept LV filling pressures low and increased LV stroke volume whereas low expression of endomyocardial NOS could have resulted in an upward shift of the diastolic LV pressure–volume relation, which increased LV filling pressures and compromised LV stroke volume.

Nitric oxide synthase and LV remodeling

NO released from the coronary endothelium provides an acute feedback between coronary perfusion and diastolic LV performance. Higher NO release from the coronary endothelium as a result of higher LV workload, higher coronary blood flow and higher coronary endothelial shear stress, optimizes LV diastolic function to accommodate the higher coronary blood flow by prolonging the diastolic time interval because of the LV relaxation-hastening effect of NO and by lowering the diastolic LV filling pressures because of the LV distensibility-increasing effect of NO. When the higher LV workload is present over an extended period of time, continuous augmentation of NO release could lead to LV dilatation and LV remodeling with return to baseline LV dimensions following cessation of the LV workload. Transient LV dilatation observed in athlete's heart could serve as an example of NO-mediated LV remodeling because in this condition coronary endothelial NO release is elevated [84] and left ventricular endomyocardial NOS gene expression upregulated [85]. The observed upregulation of endomyocardial NOS gene expression in athletes could have resulted from a myocardial stress response to repetitive exercise-related mechanical stretching. A similar upregu-

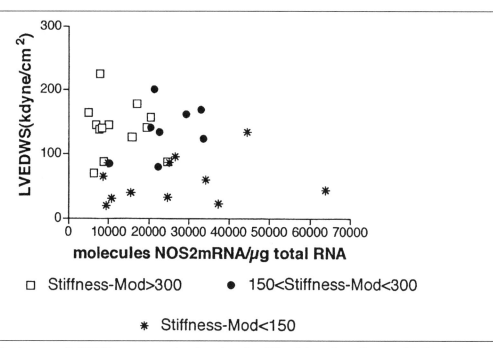

Fig. 4. *Intensity of endomyocardial NOS2 gene expression plotted against LV end-diastolic wall stress (EDWS) for different levels of LV diastolic stiffness modulus (Mod) in patients with dilated cardiomyopathy. The slope of the LVEDWS-NOS2 gene expression relation varies with the different levels of LV diastolic stiffness-Mod.*

lation of endomyocardial expression of atrial natriuretic peptide was observed in rats subjected to repetitive daily episodes of treadmill running [86] and intracoronary infusions of brain natriuretic peptide have also been demonstrated to acutely improve diastolic LV function [87].

The observed upregulation of NOS and atrial natriuretic peptide during exercise-induced LV dilatation suggests an important role for cyclic GMP, the second mediator of both NO and atrial natriuretic peptide, in physiological LV dilatation and remodeling (Fig. 5). Other myocardial signaling pathways also seem to converge on cyclic GMP such as signaling mediated by angiotensin II type 2 receptor or bradykinin type 2 receptor. Reduced NO bioavailability because of simultaneous upregulation of superoxide anion production by NADH/NADPH oxidase or because of simultaneous downregulation of antioxidant enzymes such as superoxide dismutase, catalase or hemoxygenase could result in pathological LV remodeling. In rats, chronic NOS inhibition indeed resulted in LV shrinkage with decreased LV chamber dimensions relative to wall thickness [88]. In a guinea-pig pressure-overload model, coronary endothelial stimulation with substance P no longer elicited NO-mediated LV relaxation-hastening and distensibility-increasing effects [89] probably because of angiotensin II-induced upregulation of NADH/NADPH oxidase-depen-

dent superoxide anion production [90]. Similar upregulation of NADH/NADPH oxidase with a concomitant reduction in endothelium-dependent coronary vasodilation has also been observed in post-infarct LV remodeling [91] and reacted favourably to chronic captopril treatment [48]. The deleterious effect on LV remodeling of augmented superoxide anion production could be counteracted by increased expression of anti-oxidative enzymes. In human dilated cardiomyopathy, catalase gene expression has recently been reported to be upregulated [92] and in the same patient population a coordinated expression of heme oxygenase-1 and of NOS was recently observed (Fig. 6). This coordinated expression correlated directly with LV stroke work and inversely with LV stiffness. Coordination of induction of NOS and of antioxidative enzymes probably varies in accordance to the stimulus imposed upon the myocardium. Elevation of shear stress is a well recognised stimulus for induction of heme oxygenase-1 in vascular tissue. Elevation of LV end-diastolic wall stress could therefore result in a more coordinated expression of NOS and of heme oxygenase-1 than exposure to neurohormones or to cytokines. In fact, superoxide anion-related formation of peroxynitrite and peroxynitrite-related cardio-depression have usually been reported following cytokine-induced NOS gene expression [93].

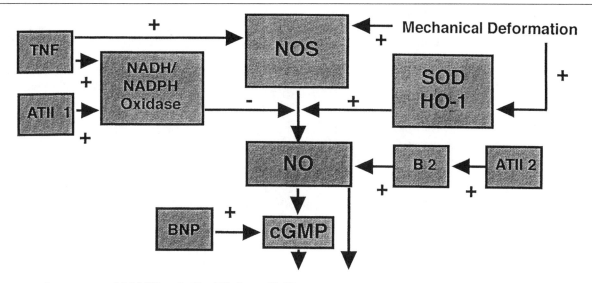

Increased LV Diastolic Distensibility and Increased LV Preload Reserve

Fig. 5. *Effects of NO on LV remodeling. NO increases diastolic LV distensibility probably through direct effects and through cGMP. Brain natriuretic peptide (BNP), angiotensin II type 2 receptor stimulation and bradykinin 2 receptor stimulation could exert similar effects on LV diastolic distensibility. Endomyocardial NO content depends on NOS activity, activity of antioxidative enzymes (SOD = Super Oxide Dismutase; HO-1 = Heme Oxygenase 1) and superoxide production by NADH/NADPH oxidase which is stimulated by angiotension II type 1 receptor stimulation or by Tumor Necrosis Factor α (TNF). Myocardial mechanical deformation because of elevated LV wall stress could lead to more coordinated upregulation of NOS and antioxidative enzymes than cytokin-mediated stimulation.*

Nitric oxide synthase and diastolic heart failure

Reduced endothelial NO production could decrease diastolic LV distensibility and could contribute to diastolic heart failure observed in the elderly, in LV hypertrophy, in diabetes, in the cardiac allograft and in ischemic heart disease. In all these conditions there is a reduction in LV distensibility paralleled by a reduction in coronary endothelial NO release.

In patients with aortic stenosis and severe LV hypertrophy, intracoronary administration of nitroglycerin or of sodium nitroprusside resulted in a marked fall in LV end-diastolic pressure and in LV end-diastolic chamber stiffness [5]. The fall observed in LV end-diastolic pressure in patients with LV hypertrophy of aortic stenosis (-39%) was larger than the fall observed in normal controls (-21%). These data suggested a higher susceptibility of hypertophied myocardium to the distensibility-increasing effect of NO. In a similar

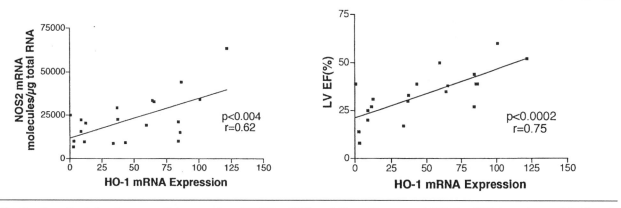

Fig. 6. *Coordinated endomyocardial expression of NOS2 mRNA and Heme Oxygenase 1(HO-1) mRNA in patients with dilated cardiomyopathy (left hand panel). Linear correlation between LV ejection fraction (EF) and HO-1 mRNA in patients with dilated cardiomyopathy (right hand panel).*

guinea-pig model of compensated LV hypertrophy induced by aortic banding, there was mild diastolic dysfunction as evident from elevation of LV end-diastolic pressure but no difference in the response of diastolic LV function to NO synthase inhibition compared to sham animals [89]. More studies are therefore needed to confirm whether hypertrophied myocardium has a truly different sensitivity to the distensibility-increasing action of NO and whether this difference results from a different baseline concentration of cyclicGMP [94] or from a different baseline concentration of cyclicAMP, which changes the susceptibility of the myocardium to the actions of cyclicGMP inhibited or cyclicGMP stimulated cyclicAMP phosphodiesterase.

The myocardial contractile effects of NO were also investigated in transplant recipients free of rejection or graft vasculopathy [2]. Compared to control subjects, transplant recipients had smaller reductions in LV peak-systolic pressure and in LV end-diastolic pressure and a similar rise in LV end-diastolic volume during bicoronary infusion of sodium nitroprusside. The fall in LV peak-systolic pressure was inversely related to measures of baseline diastolic LV function such as LV end-diastolic pressure. Baseline diastolic LV dysfunction of the cardiac allograft predicted a smaller distensibility-increasing effect of exogenous NO. Possible explanations for a reduced distensibility-increasing effect of NO in transplant recipients could be the presence of rejection-related oxidants and low baseline myocardial concentration of cyclicGMP or of cyclicAMP. In the cardiac allograft, low baseline myocardial cyclicGMP concentration could result from reduced coronary endothelial NO release because of graft vascular disease and could explain the characteristically small LV cavity size of transplanted hearts in analogy to the shrunken left ventricle of rats treated with NOS inhibitors [88]. In isolated cardiac muscle strips, the relaxation-hastening effect observed for the same dose of NO is larger at higher baseline cyclicGMP or cyclicAMP levels [94]. The smaller relaxation-hastening effect of NO in transplant recipients could therefore result not only from low baseline myocardial cyclicGMP because of coronary endothelial dysfunction but also from low baseline myocardial cyclicAMP because of cardiac denervation. In allograft recipients, the relaxation hastening effect of NO can indeed be drastically augmented following pretreatment with dobutamine [8]. Moreover, in allograft recipients with higher NOS2 gene expression in simultaneously procured endomyocardial biopsies, a dobutamine infusion elicited a larger relaxation-hastening effect and a larger reduction in peak and end-systolic LV pressures [69].

Patients with ischemic cardiomyopathy have higher LV end-diastolic pressures at comparable LV end-diastolic volumes than patients with nonischemic dilated cardiomyopathy [95]. Apart from structural differences such as scar tissue and fibrosis, reduced endothelial NO release from the atherosclerotic coronary vessels could have contributed to this decrease in LV distensibility.

Conclusions

NO has effects on contractility, energetics, apoptosis and gene expression of failing myocardium. In dilated nonischaemic cardiomyopathy, LV endomyocardial NOS gene expression is altered. Because of lower LV endomyocardial NOS gene expression in patients with higher NYHA class and lower LV stroke work, upregulated LV endomyocardial NOS gene expression seems to be beneficial rather than detrimental for failing myocardium. A beneficial effect of increased LV endomyocardial NOS gene expression could result from NO's ability to increase LV diastolic distensibility, to augment LV preload reserve, to reduce myocardial oxygen consumption and to prevent downregulation of calcium ATPase. Reduced LV endomyocardial NO content because of decreased NO or increased superoxide production could be especially important to diastolic heart failure. In many conditions such as aging, hypertension, diabetes or posttransplantation, the increased incidence of diastolic heart failure is indeed paralleled by reduced endothelium-dependent vasodilation.

References

1. Kelly RA, Han X. Nitrovasodilators have (small) direct effects on cardiac contractility. Is this important? *Circulation* 1997;96:2493–2495.
2. Paulus WJ. Nitric oxide and cardiac contraction: clinical studies. In: Lewis MJ, Shah AM, eds. *Endothelial modulation of cardiac function*. Amsterdam: Harwood academic publishers, 1997:35–51.
3. Brady AJ, Warren JB, Poole-Wilson PA, Williams TJ, Harding SE. Nitric oxide attenuates cardiac myocyte contraction. *Am J Physiol* 1993;265:H176–H182.
4. Paulus WJ, Vantrimpont PJ, Shah AM. Acute effects of nitric oxide on left ventricular relaxation and diastolic distensibility in humans. *Circulation* 1994;89:2070–2078.
5. Matter CM, Mandinov L, Kaufmann PA, Vassalli G, Jiang Z, Hess OM. Effects of NO-donors on LV diastolic function in patients with severe pressure-overload hypertrophy. *Circulation* 1999;99:2396–2401.
6. Hare JM, Loh E, Creager MA, Colucci WS. Nitric oxide inhibits the positive inotropic response to β-adrenergic stimulation in humans with left ventricular dysfunction. *Circulation* 1995;92:2198–2203.

7. Paulus WJ, Vantrimpont PJ, Shah AM. Paracrine coronary endothelial control of left ventricular function in humans. *Circulation* 1995;92:2119–2126.

8. Bartunek J, Shah AM, Vanderheyden M, Paulus WJ. Dobutamine enhances cardiodepressant effects of receptor-mediated coronary endothelial stimulation. *Circulation* 1997;95:90–96.

9. Hare JM, Givertz MM, Creager MA, Colucci WS. Increased sensitivity to nitric oxide synthase inhibition in patients with heart failure: potentiation of β-adrenergic inotropic responsiveness. *Circulation* 1998;97:161–166.

10. Shinke T, Takaoka H, Takeuchi M, Hata K, Kawai H, Okubo H, Kijima Y, Murata T, Yokoyama M. Nitric oxide spares myocardial oxygen consumption through attenuation of contractile response to β-adrenergic stimulation in patients with idiopathic dilated cardiomyopathy. *Circulation* 2000;101:1925–1930.

11. Smith JA, Shah AM, Lewis MJ. Factors released from endothelium of the ferret and pig modulate myocardial contraction. *Journal of Physiology (London)* 1991;439:1–14.

12. Meulemans AL, Sipido KR, Sys SU, Brutsaert DL. Atriopeptin III induces early relaxation of isolated mammalian papillary muscle. *Circ Res* 1988;62:1171–1174.

13. Ito N, Bartunek J, Spitzer KW, Lorell BH. Effects of the nitric oxide donor sodium nitroprusside on intercellular pH and contraction in hypertrophied myocytes. *Circulation* 1997;95:2303–2311.

14. Shah AM, Spurgeon HA, Sollott SJ, Talo A, Lakatta EG. 8-Bromo-cGMP reduces the myofilament response to Ca^{2+} in intact cardiac myocytes. *Circ Res* 1994;74:970–978.

15. Lew WYW, Ryan J, Yasuda S. Lipopolysaccharide induces cell shrinkage in rabbit ventricular cardiac myocytes. *Am J Physiol* 1997;272:H2989–H2993.

16. Clemo HF, Baumgarten CM. cGMP and atrial natriuretic factor regulate cell volume of rabbit atrial myocytes. *Circ Res* 1995;77:741–749.

17. Sagach VF, Shimanskaya TV, Sagach VV, Bogomolets AA. Coronary endothelium dysfunction and heart failure. *The Journal of Heart Failure* 1998;5:79(Abstract).

18. Prendergast BD, Sagach VF, Shah AM. Basal release of nitric oxide augments the Frank-Starling response in the isolated heart. *Circulation* 1997;96:1320–1329.

19. Pinsky DJ, Patton S, Mesaros S, Brovkovych V, Kubaszewski E, Grunfeld S, Malinski T. Mechanical transduction of nitric oxide synthesis in the beating heart. *Circ Res* 1997;81:372–379.

20. Matsubara BB, Matsubara LS, Zornoff AM, Franco M, Janicki JS. Left ventricular adaptation to chronic pressure overload induced by inhibition of nitric oxide synthase in rats. *Basic Res Cardiol* 1998;93:173–181.

21. Heymes C, Vanderheyden M, Bronzwaer JGF, Shah AM, Paulus WJ. Endomyocardial nitric oxide synthase and left ventricular preload reserve in dilated cardiomyopathy. *Circulation* 1999;99:3009–3016.

22. Recchia FA, McConnell PL, Bernstein RD, Vogel TR, Xu X, Hintze TH. Reduced nitric oxide production and altered myocardial metabolism during the decompensation of pacing-induced heart failure in the conscious dog. *Circ Res* 1998;83:969–979.

23. Gross WL, Bak MI, Ingwall JS, Arstall MA, Smith TW, Balligand JL, Kelly RA. Nitric oxide inhibits creatine kinase and regulates rat heart contractile reserve. *Proc Natl Acad Sci USA* 1996;931:5604–5609.

24. Tian R, Ingwall JS. The molecular energetics of the failing heart from animal models. *Heart Failure Reviews* 1999;4:245–253.

25. Shen W, Xu X, Ochoa M, Zhao G, Wolin MS, Hintze TH. Role of nitric oxide in the regulation of oxygen consumption in conscious dogs. *Circ Res* 1994;75:1086–1095.

26. Loke KE, Laycock SK, Mital S, Wolin MS, Bernstein R, Oz M, Addonizio L, Kaley G, Hintze TH. Nitric oxide modulates mitochondrial respiration in failing human heart. *Circulation* 1999;100:1291–1297.

27. Oddis CV, Finkel MS. Cytokine-stimulated nitric oxide production inhibits mitochondrial activity in cardiac myocytes. *Biochem Biophys Res Commun* 1995;213:1002–1009.

28. Oral H, Mann DL. Sfingosine mediates the immediate negative inotropic effects of tumor necrosis factor-alpha in the adult mammalian cardiac myocyte. *J Biol Chem* 1997;272:4836–4842.

29. Gudz TI, Tserng KY, Hoppel CL. Direct inhibition of mitochondrial respiratory chain complex III by cell-permeable ceramide. *J Biol Chem* 1997;272:24154–24158.

30. Tada H, Thompson CI, Recchia FA, Loke KE, Ochoa M, Smith CJ, Shesely EG, Kaley G, Hintze TH. Myocardial glucose uptake is regulated by nitric oxide via endothelial nitric oxide synthase in Langendorff mouse heart. *Circ Res* 2000;86:270–274.

31. Narula J, Haider N, Virmani R, Di Salvo TG, Kolodgie FD, Hajjar RJ, Schmidt U, Semigran MJ, Dec GW, Khaw BA. Apoptosis in myocytes in end-stage heart failure. *N Engl J Med* 1996;335:1182–1189.

32. Olivetti G, Abbi R, Quaini F, Kajstura J, Cheng W, Nitahara JA, Quaini E, Di Loreto C, Beltrami CA, Krajewski S, Reed JC, Anversa P. Apoptosis in the failing human heart. *N Engl J Med* 1997;336:1131–1141.

33. Schaper J, Elsässer A, Kostin S. The role of cell death in heart failure. *Circ Res* 1999;85:867–869.

34. Kim YM, Bombeck CA, Billiar TR. Nitric oxide as a bifunctional regulator of apoptosis. *Circ Res* 1999;84:253–256.

35. Koglin J, Granville DJ, Glysing-Jensen T, Mudgett JS, Carthy CM, McManus BM, Russell ME. Attenuated acute cardiac rejection in NOS2 -/- recipients correlates with reduced apoptosis. *Circulation* 1999;99:836–842.

36. Arstall MA, Sawyer DB, Fukazawa R, Kelly RA. Cytokin-mediated apoptosis in cardiac myocytes: the role of inducible nitric oxide synthase induction and peroxynitrite generation. *Circ Res* 1999;85:829–840.

37. Ing DJ, Zang J, Dzau VJ, Webster KA, Bishopric NH. Modulation of cytokine-induced cardiac myocyte apoptosis by nitric oxide, Bak, and Bcl-x. *Circ Res* 1999;84:21–33.

38. Andrew PJ, Mayer B. Enzymatic functions of nitric oxide synthases. *Cardiovascular Research* 1999;43: 521–531.

39. Ronson RS, Thourani VH, Ma XL, Katzmark SL, Han D, Zhao ZQ, Nakamura M, Guyton RA, Vinten-Johansen J. Peroxynitrite, the breakdown product of nitric oxide, is beneficial in blood cardioplegia but injurious in crystalloid cardioplegia. *Circulation* 1999;100(Suppl II):II-384–II-391.

40. Agnoletti L, Curello S, Bachetti T, Malacarne F, Gaia G, Comini L, Volterrani M, Bonetti P, Parrinello G, Cadei M, Grigolato PG, Ferrari R. Serum from patients with severe heart failure downregulates eNOS and is proapoptotic. Role of tumor necrosis factor-α. *Circulation* 1999;100:1983–1991.

41. Calderone A, Thaik CM, Takahashi N, Chang DLF, Colucci WS. Nitric oxide, atrial natriuretic peptide, and cyclic GMP inhibit the growth-promoting effects of norepinephrine in cardiac myocytes and fibroblasts. *J Clin Invest* 1998;101:812–818.

42. Barry WH. Molecular Inotropy. A future approach to the treatment of heart failure? *Circulation* 1999;100: 2303–2304.

43. Hilfiker-Kleiner D, Hilfiker A, Fehse F, Schieffer B, Harringer W, Drexler H. Endotoxin and pro-inflammatory cytokines impair α-MHC and MCK expression in cardiamyocytes in part by an E-box dependent mechanism. *Circulation* 1999;100:I-478(Abstract).

44. Bia BL, Cassidy PJ, Young ME, Rafael JA, Leighton B, Davies KE, Radda GK, Clarke K. Decreased myocardial nNOS, increased iNOS and abnormal ECG's in mouse models of Duchenne muscular dystrophy. *J Mol Cell Cardiol* 1999;31:1857–1862.

45. Badorff C, Lee GH, Lamphear BJ, Martone ME, Campbell KP, Rhoads RE, Knowlton KU. Enteroviral protease 2A cleaves dystrophin: evidence of cytoskeletal disruption in an acquired cardiomyopathy. *Nat Med* 1999;5:320–326.

46. Brahmajothi MV, Campbell DL. Heterogeneous basal expression of nitric oxide synthase and superoxide dismutase isoforms in mammalian heart. *Circ Res* 1999;85:575–587.

47. O'Murchu B, Miller VM, Perrella MA, Burnett JC Jr. Increased production of nitric oxide in coronary arteries during congestive heart failure. *J Clin Invest* 1994;93:165–171.

48. Qi XL, Stewart DJ, Gosselin H, Azad A, Picard P, Andries L, Sys SU, Brutsaert DL, Rouleau JL. Improvement of endocardial and vascular endothelial function on myocardial performance by captopril treatment in postinfarct rat hearts. *Circulation* 1999;100:1338–1345.

49. Treasure CB, Vita JA, Cox DA et al. Endothelium-dependent dilation of the coronary microvasculature is impaired in dilated cardiomyopathy. *Circulation* 1990;81:772–779.

50. Mancini GBJ, Henry GC, Macaya C, O'Neill BJ, Pucillo AL, Carere RG, Wargovich TJ, Mudra H, Lüscher TF, Klibaner MI, Haber HE, Uprichard ACG, Pepine CJ, Pitt B. Angiotensin-converting enzyme inhibition with quinapril improves endothelial vasomotor dysfunction in patients with coronary artery disease. The TREND Study. *Circulation* 1996;94:258–265.

51. Drexler H, Kästner S, Strobel A, Studer R, Brodde OE, Hasenfuss G. Expression, activity and functional significance of inducible nitric oxide synthase in the failing human heart. *J Am Coll Cardiol* 1998;32:955–963.

52. Fukuchi M, Hussain SNA, Giaid A. Heterogeneous expression and activity of endothelial and inducible nitric oxide synthase in end-stage human heart failure. Their relation to lesion site and β-adrenergic receptor therapy. *Circulation* 1998;98:132–139.

53. Stein B, Eschenhagen T, Rüdiger J, Scholz H, Förstermann U, Gath I. Increased expression of constitutive nitric oxide synthase III, but not inducible nitric oxide synthase II, in human heart failure. *J Am Coll Cardiol* 1998;32:1179–1186.

54. Nava E, Noll G, Lüscher TF. Increased activity of constitutive nitric oxide synthase in cardiac endothelium in spontaneous hypertension. *Circulation* 1995;91:2310–2313.

55. Belhassen L, Kelly RA, Smith TW, Balligand JL. Nitric Oxide Synthase (NOS3) and contractile responsiveness to adrenergic and cholinergic agonists in the heart. *J Clin Invest* 1996;97:1908–1915.

56. Belhassen L, Feron O, Kaye DM, Michel T, Kelly RA. Regulation by cAMP of post-translational processing and subcellular targeting of endothelial nitric-oxide synthase (Type 3) in cardiac myocytes. *J Biol Chem* 1997;272:11198–11204.

57. Schulz R, Nava E, Moncada S. Induction and biological relevance of a Ca^{++}-independent nitric oxide synthase in the myocardium. *Br J Pharmacol* 1992;105:575–580.

58. Finkel MS, Oddis CV, Jacob TD, Watkins SC, Hattler BG, Simmons RL. Negative inotropic effects of cytokines on the heart mediated by nitric oxide. *Science* 1992;257:387–389.

59. Yokoyama T, Vaca L, Rossen RD, Durante W, Hazarika P, Mann DL. Cellular basis for the negative inotropic effects of tumor necrosis factor-α in the adult mammalian heart. *J Clin Invest* 1993;92:2303–2312.

60. Hirono S, Islam MO, Nakazawa M, Yoshida Y, Kodama M, Shibata A, Izumi T, Imai S. Expression of inducible nitric oxide synthase in rat experimental autoimmune myocarditis with special reference to changes in cardiac hemodynamics. *Circ Res* 1997;80:11–20.

61. Wang WZ, Matsumori A, Yamada T, Shioi T, Okada I, Matsui S, Sato Y, Suzuki H, Shiota K, Sasayama S. Beneficial effects of amlodipine in a murine model of congestive heart failure induced by viral myocarditis. *Circulation* 1997;95:245–251.

62. MacMicking JD, Nathan C, Hom G, Chartrain N, Fletcher DS, Trumbauer M, Stevens K, Xie Q, Sokol K, Hutchinson N, Chen H, Mudgett JS. Altered responses to bacterial infection and endotoxic shock in mice lacking inducible nitric oxide synthase. *Cell* 1995;81:641–650.

63. Pagani FD, Baker LS, Hsi C, Knox M, Fink MP, Visner MS. Left ventricular systolic and diastolic dysfunction after infusion of tumor necrosis factor-α in conscious dogs. *J Clin Invest* 1992;90:389–398.

64. Murray DR, Freeman GL. Tumor necrosis factor-α induces a biphasic effect on myocardial contractility in conscious dogs. *Circ Res* 1996;78:154–160.

65. Yamamoto S, Tsutsui H, Tagawa H, Saito K, Takahashi M, Tada H, Yamamoto M, Katoh M, Egashira K, Takeshita A. Role of myocyte nitric oxide in β-adrenergic hyporesponsiveness in heart failure. *Circulation* 1997;95:1111–1114.

66. de Belder AJ, Radomski M, Why H, Richardson PJ, Bucknall CA, Salas E, Martin JF. Nitric oxide synthase activities in human myocardium. *Lancet* 1993;341:84–85.

67. Lewis NP, Tsao PS, Rickenbacher PR, Xue C, Johns RA, Haywood GA, von der Leyen H, Trindade PT, Cooke JP, Hunt SA, Billingham ME, Valantine HA, Fowler MB. Induction of nitric oxide synthase in the human allograft is associated with contractile dysfunction of the left ventricle. *Circulation* 1996;93:720–729.

68. Haywood GA, Tsao PS, von der Leyen HE, Mann MJ, Keeling PJ, Trindade PT, Lewis NP, Byrne CD, Rickenbacher PR, Bishopric NH, Cooke JP, McKenna WJ, Fowler MB. Expression of inducible nitric oxide synthase in human heart failure. *Circulation* 1996;93:1087–1094.

69. Paulus WJ, Kästner S, Pujadas P, Shah AM, Drexler H, Vanderheyden M. Left ventricular contractile effects of inducible nitric oxide synthase in the human allograft. *Circulation* 1997;96:3436–3442.

70. Satoh M, Nakamura M, Tamura G, Makita S, Segawa I, Tashiro A, Satodate R, Hiramori K. Inducible nitric oxide synthase and tumor necrosis factor-alpha in myocardium in human dilated cardiomyopathy. *J Am Coll Cardiol* 1997;29:716–724.

71. Oddis CV, Simmons RL, Hattler BG, Finkel MS. cAMP enhances inducible nitric oxide synthase mRNA stability in cardiac myocytes. *Am J Physiol* 1995;269:H2044–H2050.

72. Pinsky DJ, Cai B, Yang X, Rodriguez C, Sciacca RR, Cannon PJ. The lethal effects of cytokine-induced nitric oxide on cardiac myocytes are blocked by nitric oxide synthase antagonism or transforming growth factor β. *J Clin Invest* 1995;95:677–685.

73. Inoue N, Venema RC, Sayegh HS et al. Molecular regulation of the bovine endothelial cell nitric oxide synthase by transforming growth factor-beta 1. *Arterioscler Thromb Vasc Biol* 1995;15:1255–1261.

74. Taketani S, Sawa Y, Taniguchi K et al. C-Myc expression and its role in patients with chronic aortic regurgitation. *Circulation* 1997;96:II-83–II-89.

75. Hirota H, Chen J, Betz UA et al. Loss of gp130 cardiac muscle cell survival pathway is a critical event in the onset of heart failure during biomechanical stress. *Cell* 1999;97:189–198.

76. Li YY, Feldman AM, Sun Y, McTiernan CF. Differential expression of tissue inhibitors of metalloproteinases in the failing human heart. *Circulation* 1998;98:1728–1734.

77. Spinale FG, Coker ML, Krombach SR, Mukherjee R, Hallak H, Houck WV, Clair MJ, Kribbs SB, Johnson LJ, Peterson JT, Zile MR. Matrix metalloproteinase inhibition during the development of congestive heart failure. Effects on left ventricular dimensions and function. *Circ Res* 1999;85:364–376.

78. Mann DL, Spinale FG. Activation of matrix metalloproteinases in the failing human heart. Breaking the tie that binds. *Circulation* 1998;98:1699–1702.

79. Higginbotham MB, Sullivan MJ, Coleman RE, Cobb FR. Regulation of stroke volume during exercise in patients with severe left ventricular dysfunction: Importance of the Starling mechanism. *J Am Coll Cardiol* 1987;9:58.

80. Holubarsch C, Ruf T, Goldstein DJ, Ashton RC, Nickl W, Pieske B, Pioch K, Lüdemann J, Wiesner S, Hasenfuss G, Posival H, Just H, Burkhoff D. Existence of the Frank-Starling mechanism in the failing human heart. *Circulation* 1996;94:683–689.

81. Pinamonti B, Di Lenarda A, Sinagra GF, Camerini F and the Heart Muscle Disease Study Group. Restrictive left ventricular filling pattern in dilated cardiomyopathy assessed by Doppler echocardiography: Clinical, echocardiographic and hemodynamic correlations and prognostic implications. *J Am Coll Cardiol* 1993;22:808–815.

82. Rihal CS, Nishimura RA, Hatle LK, Bailey KR, Tajik AJ. Systolic and diastolic dysfunction in patients with clinical diagnosis of dilated cardiomyopathy: relation to symptoms and prognosis. *Circulation* 1994;90:2772–2779.

83. Zeitz CJ, Bronzwaer JGF, Heymes C, Vanderheyden M, Paulus WJ. Left ventricular end-diastolic wall stress and endomyocardial inducible nitric oxide syntase gene expression in human dilated cardiomyopathy. *J Am Coll Cardiol* 2000;35:204(Abstract).

84. Wang J, Wolin MS, Hintze TH. Chronic exercise enhances endothelium-mediated dilation of epicardial coronary artery in conscious dogs. *Circ Res* 1993;73:829–838.

85. Sessa WC, Pritchard K, Seyedi N, Wang J, Hintze TH. Chronic exercise in dogs increases coronary vascular nitric oxide production and endothelial cell nitric oxide synthase gene expression. *Circ Res* 1994;74:349–353.

86. Mantymaa P, Arokoski J, Porsti I, Perhonen M, Arvola P, Helminen HJ, Takala TE, Leppaluoto J, Ruskoaho H. Effect of endurance training on atrial natriuretic peptide gene expression in normal and hypertrophied hearts. *J Appl Physiol* 1994;76:1184–1194.

87. Yamamoto K, Burnett JC Jr, Redfield MM. Effect of endogenous natriuretic peptide system on ventricular and coronary function in failing heart. *Am J Physiol* 1997;273:H2406–H2414.

88. Bartunek J, Weinberg EO, Tajima M, Rohrbach S, Katz SE, Douglas PS, Lorell BH. Chronic L-NAME-induced hypertension: novel molecular adaptation to systolic load in absence of hypertrophy. *Circulation* 2000;101:423–429.

89. MacCarthy PA, Shah AM. Impaired endothelium-dependent regulation of ventricular relaxation in pressure-overload cardiac hypertrophy. *Circulation* 2000;101:1854–1860.

90. Lang D, Mosfer SI, Shakesby A, Donaldson F, Lewis MJ. Coronary microvascular endothelial cell redox state in left ventricular hypertrophy. The role of angiotensin II. *Circ Res* 2000;86:463–469.

91. Bauersachs J, Bouloumié A, Fraccarollo D, Hu K, Busse R, Ertl G. Endothelial dysfunction in chronic myocardial infarction despite increased vascular endothelial nitric oxide synthase and soluble guanylate cyclase expression: role of enhanced vascular superoxide production. *Circulation* 1999;100:292–298.

92. Dieterich S, Bieligk U, Beulich K, Hasenfuss G, Prestle J. Gene expression of antioxidative enzymes in the human heart. *Circulation* 2000;101:33–39.

93. Panas D, Khadow FH, Szabo C, Schulz R. Proinflammatory cytokines depress cardiac efficiency by nitric oxide dependent mechanism. *Am J Physiol* 1998;275:H1016–H1023.

94. Mohan P, Brutsaert DL, Paulus WJ, Sys SU. Myocardial contractile response to nitric oxide and cGMP. 1996;93:1223–1229.

95. Hare JM, Walford GD, Hruban RH, Hutchins GM, Deckers JW, Baugham KL. Ischemic cardiomyopathy: endomyocardial biopsy and ventriculographic evaluation of patients with congestive heart failure, dilated cardiomyopathy and coronary artery disease. *J Am Coll Cardiol* 1992;20:1318–1325.

6. Interactions Between Cytokines and Neurohormonal Systems in the Failing Heart

Hong Kan, MD, PhD[1] and
Mitchell S. Finkel, MD[1,2]

[1]Departments of Medicine (Cardiology), [2]Pharmacology and Toxicology, West Virginia University School of Medicine, Robert C. Byrd Health Sciences Center, Louis A. Johnson V.A. Medical Center, Morgantown, WV 26506-9157.

Introduction

Congestive heart failure (CHF) remains an enormous health care problem in the United States, as well as other industrialized countries [1–3]. Millions of Americans are currently being treated for CHF and hundreds of thousands of others are expected to join their ranks annually. The prognosis for CHF patients has been improved as a result of the use of angiotensin converting enzyme inhibitors (ACEI) and β-adrenergic receptor blockers (β-blockers) [1–4]. The success of these therapies underscores the pathogenic role of neurohormonal activation in CHF. It is now widely appreciated that norepinephrine (NE) and angiotensin II (AII) directly contribute to progressive deterioration in myocardial function and are not merely markers of disease severity or epiphenomenae [5–7].

A role for the immune system in the regulation of myocardial function in CHF has also been proposed [8]. Insights derived from clinical and basic studies into the myocardial effects of sepsis were critical to achieving this understanding. The existence of a 'circulating myocardial depressant factor' was first proposed to explain the reversible myocardial depression observed clinically in patients with sepsis [9]. Subsequently, plasma levels of pro-inflammatory cytokines were found to be elevated in patients with sepsis and anti-cytokine antibodies were reported to reverse sepsis-induced myocardial depression in patients [10–12].

Other clinical observations appear to support a similar pathophysiologic role for cytokines in CHF. Elevated circulating levels of the pro-inflammatory cytokine, tumor necrosis factor alpha (TNF) have been independently associated with a worse prognosis in CHF [13]. The adverse impact of increased cytokine levels is reminiscent of the earlier association of elevated NE levels with a poor prognosis in CHF [5]. In addition, transgenic overexpression of TNF alone has been reported to be sufficient to induce a CHF phenotype in a rodent [14]. Thus, the elaboration of cytokines along with AII and NE appear to play an important role in the progressive deterioration that is a hallmark of chronic heart failure. This review will focus on the relationship between neurohormonal and immune responses to myocardial injury in CHF. A novel hypothesis is proposed to explain the reversible component of myocardial dysfunction and β-adrenergic desensitization seen in CHF, based on insights derived from the reversible myocardial dysfunction and β-adrenergic desensitization associated with ischemia and sepsis.

Reversible myocardial effects of ischemia and sepsis

Myocardial ischemia followed by reperfusion was first shown to be associated with a transient period of depressed contractility in the opened chest dog model [6]. The clinical implications of these experimental observations were not fully appreciated until sophisticated imaging techniques enabled clinicians to assess myocardial contractility and viability non-invasively in patients [15]. It has become increasingly apparent that a number of clinical conditions result in reversible depression of myocardial contractility. Reversible myocardial depression following reperfusion of ischemic myocardium has been documented in patients following myocardial infarction, cardiopulmonary bypass, thrombolytic therapy and coronary angioplasty [15]. This phenomenon is generally referred to as myocardial 'stunning'.

A number of non-ischemic conditions have also been shown to be associated with reversible myocardial depression in animal models and humans. The systemic inflammatory response syndrome (SIRS) seen in sepsis is one such condition that may serve as a paradigm for reversible myocardial depression associated with both ischemic and non-ischemic etiologies. The myocardial effects of sepsis have three characteristics shared by myocardial ischemia, and congestive heart failure:

Douglas L. Mann. THE ROLE OF INFLAMMATORY MEDIATORS IN THE FAILING HEART.
Copyright © 2001. Kluwer Academic Publishers. Boston. All rights reserved.

(1) activation of inflammatory mediators
(2) reversible myocardial depression
(3) β-adrenergic desensitization [9–11,16,17].

The reversible myocardial depression and β-adrenergic desensitization seen in these conditions can be explained on the basis of effects of cytokine induced nitric oxide (NO) production. Considerable evidence exists supporting a role for pro-inflammatory cytokines and nitric oxide (NO) in the regulation of myocardial function [6,12,16,18–41]. The mechanism(s) responsible for the myocardial effects of these endogenous mediators can be further explained on the basis of established principles of myocardial excitation–contraction coupling (E–C coupling).

Myocardial excitation–contraction (E–C) coupling

Depolarization of the cardiac myocyte sarcolemmal membrane during the action potential results in the intracellular entry of extracellular calcium. The major regulators of the transsarcolemmal entry of calcium include L-type calcium channels and autonomic receptors [21,42] (Fig. 1). These membrane bound proteins all contribute to the influx of a minute quantity of calcium from outside the cell into the myocyte. The small quantity of calcium that traverses the L-type calcium channel during membrane depolarization causes the release of the large reservoir of calcium stored in the sarcoplasmic reticulum (SR) through the SR calcium release channel (ryanodine receptor) (Fig. 1). This large reservoir of calcium then interacts with tropomyosin to allow the actin and myosin filaments to overlap. This results in systolic myocardial contraction. Diastolic relaxation results from the resequestration of this large reservoir of calcium back into the sarcoplasmic reticulum through the SR calcium/ATPase. Calcium exits the cell through the Na^+/Ca^{++} exchanger and sarcolemmal Ca^{++} ATPase (Fig. 1).

Autonomic receptors further regulate calcium influx through the sarcolemma (Fig. 1) [21,42]. β-adrenergic stimulation results in the association of a catalytic subunit of a G-protein coupled to the β receptor. This stimulates the enzyme, adenylate cyclase, to convert ATP to cAMP. Increasing cAMP production results in cAMP dependent phosphorylation of the L-type calcium channel. Phosphorylation results in an increase in the probability for the open state of the channel. This translates into an increase in transsarcolemmal calcium influx during phase 2 (i.e. the plateau phase) of the action potential. Alpha adrenergic receptor stimulation results in the

phospholipase C-mediated breakdown of phosphatidylcholine to inositol triphosphate (IP_3) and diacyl glycerol (DAG). These second messengers further enhance mobilization of both transsarcolemmal calcium influx and SR calcium efflux.

The mechanism by which transsarcolemmal calcium activates the release of SR calcium is not completely understood. It does appear to involve an allosteric conformational change in the SR release channel caused by the binding of calcium to a specific site [21,42]. It has been shown that sulfhydryl agents regulate calcium release from skeletal and cardiac SR vesicles [43]. The physiologic gating of the ryanodine-sensitive SR release channel appears to be dependent on the redox state of critical sulfhydryl groups residing on the SR membrane. Experimental evidence indicates that the oxidation or reduction of free sulfhydryls on the SR calcium release channel plays an important role in the reversible component of myocardial depression in the Syrian hamster cardiomyopathy model [44]. The sulfhydryl agent, acetylcysteine, reversed the depressed contractility in this animal model. This observation is particularly interesting in view of an elegant demonstration that nitric oxide can modulate cardiac SR calcium release by nitrosylation of sulfhydryls [41]. Thus, changes in NO levels within cardiac myocytes could modulate contractility by altering E–C coupling (Fig. 2).

Nitric oxide and cytokines

Nitric oxide (NO) has been reported to play a role in a wide range of cellular processes including cellular proliferation, apoptosis and mitochondrial electron transport [45] (Fig. 2). Nitric oxide is formed from the oxidation of one of the two chemically equivalent guanidino nitrogens of the amino acid, L-arginine, by a distinct family of NO synthases [10,47–50]. Two different constitutive (present all the time) (cNOS) and a single inducible (requires gene expression) (iNOS) enzymes have been cloned and sequenced [10,47–50]. cNOS's have been described in neural tissue (type I) and endothelium (type III). Cytokines induce a third type of NOS (type II). Arginine analogues such as L-NMMA block the production of NO by competitively inhibiting NO synthase enzyme activity [45]. The addition of L-arginine can overcome this inhibition [45]. NO has been shown to have a variety of effects on cardiac myocytes, including raising cGMP levels by activating soluble guanylate cyclase, inhibit mitochondrial electron transport, reduce affinity of contractile proteins for calcium, decrease transsarcolemmal calcium influx by phosphoryla-

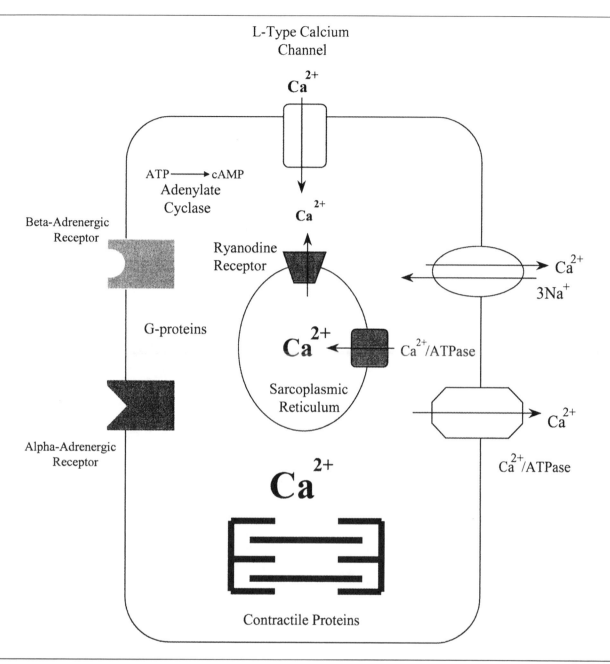

Fig. 1. *Schematic diagram illustrating the movement of calcium from the extracellular space to trigger intracellular release of calcium followed by extrusion of calcium back into the extracellular space. Calcium enters the myocyte through L-type calcium channels that are modulated by (α and β) adrenergic receptors. This small quantity of calcium triggers the release of the large reservoir of intracellular calcium stored in the SR (sarcoplasmic reticulum) by activation of the SR calcium release channel (ryanodine receptor). Calcium is resequestered into the SR by the SR calcium/ATPase. Calcium is extruded from the cell largely through the Na$^+$/Ca^{++} exchanger and the sarcolemmal calcium ATPase.*

tion of L-type calcium channels and modulate SR calcium release by s-nitrosylation (Fig. 2) [45].

Proinflammatory cytokines are a class of secretory polypeptides that are synthesized and released locally by macrophages, leukocytes and endothelial cells in response to injury [51]. Interleukins 1,6 and TNF (Tumor Necrosis Factor-α)

are cytokines that are produced by immune cells in response to challenge or injury [51]. Interleukin (IL)-2 administration to animal models and cancer patients elicited reversible hemodynamic changes similar to those seen in shock due to gram-negative bacterial sepsis [52]. Patients developed sinus tachycardia, decreased mean

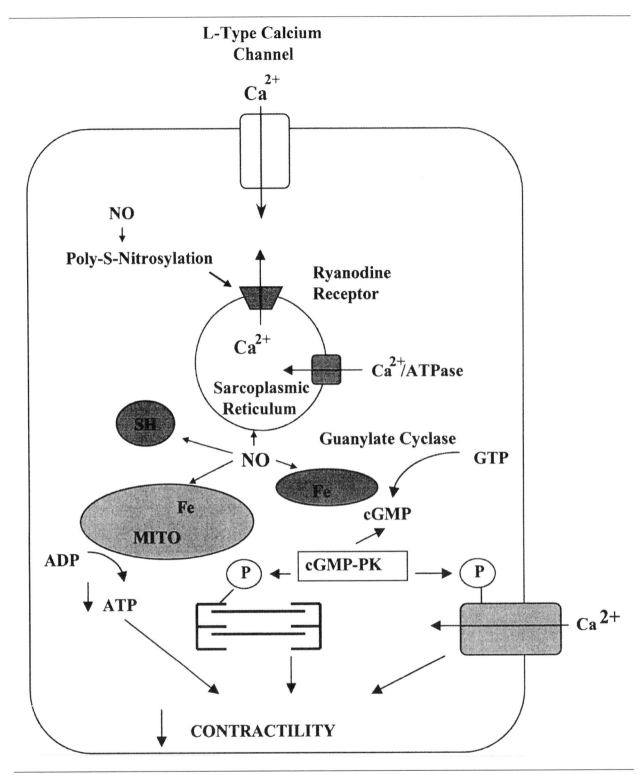

Fig. 2. *Schematic diagram illustrating potential effects of nitric oxide (NO) on cardiac myocytes. NO production activates guanylate cyclase by binding to iron which converts GTP to cGMP. cGMP can depress myocardial contractility by phosphorylating sarcolemmal L-type calcium channels and/or contractile proteins. cGMP dependent phosphorylation of calcium channels diminishes the influx of extracellular calcium while phosphorylation of contractile proteins lowers their affinity for calcium. In addition, the large quantities of NO that result from iNOS activation depress mitochondrial activity by binding to iron in succinate dehydrogenase. Depression of L-type calcium channel activity, lowering the affinity of contractile proteins for calcium and the suppression of mitochondrial activity all can contribute to depression in myocardial contractility. In addition, NO can modulate contractility by poly-s-nitrosylating the sarcoplasmic reticulum calcium release channel (Ryanodine Receptor).*

arterial pressure, increased cardiac index, decreased systemic vascular resistance and a fall in left ventricular ejection fraction.

These hemodynamic effects that are seen in sepsis from gram-negative bacteria have been attributed to endotoxin (lipopolysaccharide-LPS) in the bacterial membrane [10]. LPS has been shown to mediate effects through stimulation of mononuclear phagocytes [51]. Of the variety of mediators released by these cells, TNF, IL-1, and IL-6 appear to play a pivotal role in mediating the hemodynamic effects of gram-negative sepsis and shock [10,11,16,19,51]. TNF, IL-6, and IL-2 all reversibly depressed contractility of isolated rodent left ventricular papillary muscles [24]. The NO synthase inhibitor, L-NMMA, blocked these negative inotropic effects. L-Arginine reversed the inhibition by L-NMMA by providing additional substrate for NO production. These results suggested that the direct negative inotropic effects of cytokines on the heart were dependent on the enhanced activity of a myocardial cNOS enzyme. Subsequent molecular and cellular studies definitively demonstrated the presence of a functional cNOS (NOSIII) in cardiac myocytes [20,31]. Inflammatory cytokines have also been shown to reduce the positive inotropic response of isolated cardiac myocytes to the β-adrenergic agonist, isoproterenol, through a mechanism possibly involving NO [27,34,35,38]. TNF and IL-1 have been shown to uncouple agonist-occupied receptors from adenylate cyclase in isolated cardiac myocytes [27]. These findings implicated guanine nucleotide binding protein (G-protein) function in the direct or indirect action of cytokines on the heart. G-protein mediated depression of cardiac myocyte L-type calcium channels by IL-1 has also been reported [34]. This is consistent with a cGMP-mediated effect of NO on cardiac L-type calcium channels. Thus, β-adrenergic desensitization (hyporesposiveness) could result from a cytokine-mediated, NO dependent suppression of cardiac L-type calcium channels (Fig. 2).

The spontaneous beating rates of neonatal cardiac myocytes are also dependent on sarcolemmal L-type calcium channel activity [21,42]. Treatment of neonatal cardiac myocytes with cytokines have been reported to blunt the positive chronotropic effect of β-adrenergic stimulation with isoproterenol [53]. Thus, the regulation of the sarcolemmal L-type calcium channel could explain both the inotropic and chronotropic effects of cytokines on the heart.

Stunned myocardium

The observed direct inotropic and chronotropic effects of proinflammatory cytokines raised the possibility that they participate in reversible post-ischemic myocardial depression ('Stunned myocardium') [15]. Cardiopulmonary bypass predictably results in reversible myocardial dysfunction and β-adrenergic desensitization [54,55]. Elevated levels of IL-6 were detected in patients immediately following aortocoronary bypass grafting [26]. These same concentrations of IL-6 were also shown to reversibly depress contractility in human cardiac tissue [26]. Other laboratories have independently confirmed the presence of elevated IL-6 levels in cardiac surgical patients [54,55]. Serum IL-6 levels have also been reported to be elevated in patients and animal models following myocardial infarction [56,57]. From these observations, it is intriguing to speculate that IL-6 could contribute to the transient myocardial depression, 'stunning', that is known to occur following cardiopulmonary bypass and myocardial infarction. The potential role for NO in post-CABG myocardial stunning was further explored by assaying for its stable end-products, NO_2^- (nitrite) and NO_3^- (nitrate) [29,30]. Coronary sinus nitrite and nitrate levels were increased 10 fold in patients following coronary artery bypass surgery. In addition, NO synthase enzyme activity was increased 3 fold in pectinate muscles from these patients following the same surgery. These elevated levels of NO products were temporally associated with postoperative myocardial stunning. Taken together, these findings support a cytokine-stimulated, NO-mediated mechanism for myocardial stunning following cardiopulmonary bypass. The potential therapeutic implications of these studies justify future efforts to elucidate the molecular mechanisms involved in the effects of cytokines and NO on the heart.

Congestive heart failure

Reversible myocardial depression and β-adrenergic desensitization occurs in CHF, as well as sepsis and ischemia [9–11,16,17]. This phenomenon raises the possibility that common endogenous mediators stimulated by a variety of diverse injuries manifest a shared 'program' of responses. These programmed host responses are designed to enhance survival following hemorrhage, trauma and infection. The short-term survival benefits of AII and NE are obvious to maintain hemodynamic stability in response to hemorrhage. Unfortunately, the persistent, unrelenting, response of AII and NE in CHF confers no survival advantage and is, in fact, deleterious. This AII and NE programmed survival response to hemorrhage is also accompanied by the cytokine and NO response to infection in CHF. The triggering of these inappropriate responses is considered to be a major mechanism responsible

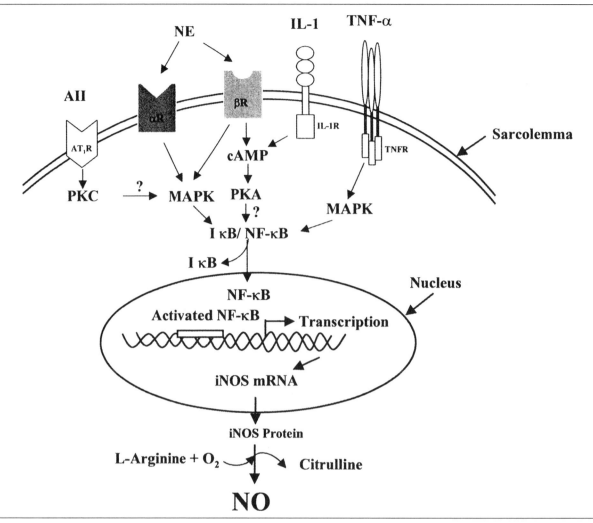

Fig. 3. *Schematic diagram illustrating the effects of the binding of interleukin 1β (IL-1) with angiotensin II (AII), norepinephrine (NE), and tumor necrosis factor α (TNF) to receptors on the surface of a cardiac myocyte. Binding of IL-1 alone to its receptor is sufficient to induce iNOS mRNA and protein synthesis over several hours. This is associated with increased cAMP formation, protein kinase A (PKA) activation, activation and nuclear translocation of nuclear factor kappa B (NFκB). Angiotensin II (AII) enhances NO production by activation of protein kinase C (PKC) and possibly mitogen activated protein kinase (MAPK). Norepinephrine (NE) binds to both α and β adrenergic receptors that activate MAPK via cAMP independent and dependent mechanisms. Tumor necrosis factor alpha (TNFα) also enhances NO production by stimulating MAPK to enhance NFκB activation and nuclear translocation. Neither AII, NE or TNFα alone can induce iNOS expression. However, all three endogenous mediators enhance IL-1 stimulated iNOS mRNA expression, iNOS protein synthesis and NO production.*

for the inexorable decline in CHF. Nitric oxide appears to play a central role in this maladaptive program.

Cytokines induce the expression of iNOS (NOS II) in cardiac myocytes [6,18,19,22,28,32,33,36, 38,40]. This revelation has now provided a novel approach to understanding the role of cytokines and NO in congestive heart failure patients (CHF). Cytokine-stimulated NO production reversibly inhibited mitochondrial enzyme activity in cardiac myocytes [6,39,40]. Angiotensin II, norepinephrine and TNF increase NO production in cardiac myocytes through different molecular mechanisms (Fig. 3) [32,33,36]. Each of these

endogenous mediators have their own cardiac receptors with distinct signaling pathways. AII has been shown to enhance cardiac myocyte NO production by stimulating protein kinase C activity [58]. NE binds to both α- and β-adrenergic receptors that directly, or indirectly stimulate mitogen activated protein kinases (MAPK) to activate nuclear factor κB (NFκB) to translocate from cytosol to the nucleus after dissociating from IκB. TNFα similarly stimulates MAPK mediated NFκB activation and nuclear translocation. Activated NFκB facilitates transcription of iNOS mRNA, followed by translation to iNOS protein and enhanced NO production by converting the amino acid, L-Arginine, to citrulline and NO. All of this fine coordination between the endocrine, autonomic and immune systems suggests an important role for NO in this maladaptive programmed host response to injury. AII, NE or TNF alone, do not increase NO. They only synergize with IL-1. This requirement for IL-1 provides added refinement and modulation of this complex system. The diversity of stimuli and/or injuries that can result in AII, NE, TNF and IL-1 elaboration suggests that this iNOS/NO response has adaptive advantages, as well.

These observations in cardiac myocytes may provide important insights into the molecular mechanisms responsible for the deleterious effects of cAMP elevating agents and the poor prognosis associated with elevated circulating levels of Angiotensin II, norepinephrine and TNF in CHF [1,5,13]. The reported improvements in both ventricular function and survival with the combined alpha and beta adrenergic receptor blocker, carvedilol, in CHF supports the clinical relevance of these *in vitro* studies [3].

Further support for the clinical relevance of NO in CHF can be found in papillary muscle studies [25]. The NO synthase inhibitor, L-NMMA, reversed the negative inotropic effect of increasing stimulation frequency in isolated hamster papillary muscles (negative force-frequency; negative 'Staircase') [25]. L-NMMA also blunted the negative inotropic effect of the sarcoplasmic reticulum calcium release channel regulator, ryanodine [25]. Papillary muscles isolated from CHF patients also demonstrate a negative force-frequency response [59]. The inotropic response of cardiac myocytes to stimulation frequency is dependent on the relationship between the sarcolemmal L-type calcium channel, sarcoplasmic reticulum calcium release channel and the Na^+/Ca^{++} exchanger (E–C coupling; Fig. 1). Cytokine-mediated, NO dependent alterations in E–C coupling could result in changes in the force–frequency relationship. Taken together, these basic and clinical observations support a pathophysiologically relevant role for cytokines and NO in CHF, as well.

Conclusions

The success of ACE inhibitors and β blockers underscores the pathogenic role of neurohormonal activation in CHF. Clinical and experimental evidence suggests a pathophysiologic role for cytokines and NO in the effects of AII and NE in CHF. The *in vitro* effects of these endogenous mediators suggest that they may contribute to the pathogenesis of the reversible myocardial depression and β-adrenergic desensitization observed clinically in patients with sepsis, ische-

mia and congestive heart failure. Basic studies of cytokine signaling pathways in cardiac myocytes have the potential to identify novel therapeutic targets for the treatment of cardiac patients.

Acknowledgments

This research was supported by the National Institutes of Health, Grant #HL-53372, American Heart Association (Ohio Valley Affiliate), the US Department of Veteran Affairs and the West Virginia University (WVU) Foundation.

References

1. The CONSENSUS Trial Study Group. Effects of enalapril on mortality in severe congestive heart failure. Results of the Cooperative North Scandinavian Enalapril Survial Study (CONSENSUS). *N Engl J Med* 1987;316:1429–1435.
2. Ho KK, Anderson KM, Kannel WB, et al. Survival after the onset of congestive heart failure in Framingham Heart Study subjects. *Circulation* 1993;88:107–115.
3. Packer M, Bristow MR, Cohn JN, et al. for the U.S. Carvedilol Heart Failure Study Group. The effect of carvedilol on morbidity and mortality in patients with chronic heart failure. *N Engl J Med* 1996;334:1349–1355.
4. Swedberg K, Hjalmarson A, Waagstein F, Wallentin I. Prolongation of survival in congestive cardiomyopathy by beta-receptor blockade. *Lancet* 1979;2:1374–1376.
5. Cohn JN, Levine TB, Olivari MT, et al. Plasma norepinephrine as a guide to prognosis in patients with chronic congestive heart failure. *N Eng J Med* 1984;311:819.
6. Oddis CV, Finkel MS. Cytokine-stimulated nitric oxide production inhibits mitochondrial activity in cardiac myocytes. *Biochem and Biophys Res Comm* 1995;213(3):1002–1009.
7. Sadoshima J, Izumo S. Signal transduction pathways of angiotension II-induced c-fos gene expression in cardiac myocytes in vitro. *Circ Res* 1993;73:424–438.
8. Mann DL, Young JB. Basic mechanisms in congestive heart failure. Recognizing the role of proinflammatory cytokines. *Chest* 1994;105:897–904.
9. Reilly JM, Cunnion RE, Burch-Whitman C, Parker MM, Shelhamer JH, Parrillo JE. A circulating myocardial depressant substance is associated with cardiac dysfunction and peripheral hypoperfusion (lactic acidemia) in patients with septic shock. *Chest* 1989;95:1072–1080.
10. Parillo JE. Mechanisms of disease: pathogenic mechanisms of septic shock. *N Eng J Med* 1993;328:1471–1477.
11. Parker MM, Shelhamer JH, Bacharach SL, Green MV, Natanson C, Frederick TM, Damske BA, Parrillo JE. Profound but reversible myocardial depression in patients with septic shock. *Annals of Internal Medicine* 1985;100:483–490.
12. Vincent JL, Bakker J, Marecaux G, Schandene L, Kahn RJ, Dupont E. Administration of anti-TNF antibody improves left ventricular function in septic shock patients. *Chest* 1992;101:810–815.
13. Levine B, Kalman J, Mayer L, Filit HM, Packer M. Elevated circulating levels of tumor necrosis factor in

severe chronic heart failure. *N Eng J Med* 1990;323(4):236–241.

14. Feldman AM, Combes A, Wagner D, Kadakomi T, Kubota T, Li YY, McTiernan C. The role of tumor necrosis factor in the pathophysiology of heart failure. *J Am Coll Cardiol* 2000;35:537–544.

15. Braunwald E, Kloner RA. The stunned myocardium: Prolonged, postischemic ventricular dysfunction. *Circulation* 1982;66:1146–1149.

16. Kumar AR, Brar R, Wang P, Dee L, Skorupa G, Khadour F, Schulz R, Parrillo JE. Role of nitric oxide and cAMP in human septic serum-induced depression of cardiac myocyte contractility. *Am J Physiol* 1999;276:R265–R276.

17. Smith LW, McDonough KH. Inotropic sensitivity to adrenergic stimulation in early sepsis. *Am J Physiol* 1988;255 (*Heart Circ. Physiol.* 24):H699–H703.

18. Balligand JL, Ungureanu-Longrois D, Simmons WW, Pimental D, Malinski TA, Kapturczak M, Taha Z, Lowenstein CJ, Davidoff AJ, Kelly RA, Smith TW, Michel T. Cytokine-inducible nitric oxide synthase (iNOS) expression in cardiac myocytes. *J Biol Chem* 1994;269:27580–27588.

19. Balligand JL, Ungureann D, Kelly RA, Kobzik L, Pimental D, Michael T, Smith TW. Abnormal contractile function due to induction of nitric oxide synthesis in rat cardiac myocytes follows exposure to activated macrophage-conditioned medium. *J Clin Invest* 1993;91:2314–2319.

20. Balligand JL, Kobzik L, Han X, Kaye DM, Belhassen L, O'Hara DS, Kelly RA, Smith TW, Michel T. Nitric oxide-dependent parasympathetic signaling is due to activation of constitutive endothelial (Type III) nitric oxide synthase in cardiac myocytes. *J Biol Chem* 1995;270(4):14582–14586.

21. Bers DM. Excitation-contraction coupling and cardiac contractile force. Norwell: Kluwer Academic Publishers, 1991:119–145.

22. Brady AJB, Warren JB, Poole-Wilson PA, Williams TJ, Harding SE. Nitric oxide attenuates cardiac myocyte contraction. *Am J Physiol* 1993;265:H176–H182.

23. Drexler H, Kastner S, Strobel A, Studer R, Brodde OE, Hasenfub G. Expression, activity and functional significance of inducible nitric oxide synthase in the failing human heart. *J Am Coll Cardiol* 1998;32:955–963.

24. Finkel MS, Oddis CV, Jacobs TD, Watkins SC, Hattler BG, Simmons RL. Inotropic effects of cytokines on the heart mediated by nitric oxide. *Science* 1992;257:387–389.

25. Finkel MS, Oddis CV, Mayer OH, Hattler BG, Simmons RL. Nitric oxide synthase inhibitor alters papillary muscle force-frequency relationship. *J Pharm Exp Ther* 1995;272(2):945–952.

26. Finkel MS, Shen L, Oddis CV, Hoffman RA, Romeo RC, Simmons RL, Hattler BG. IL-6 as a mediator of stunned myocardium. *Am J Cardiol* 1993;71:1231–1232.

27. Gulick T, Chung MK, Peiper SJ, Lange LG, Schreiner GF. Interleukin-1 and tumor necrosis factor inhibit cardiac myocytes-adrenergic responsiveness. *Proc Natl Acad Sci USA* 1989;86:6753–6757.

28. Habib FM, Spingall DR, Davies GJ, Oakley CM, Yacoub MH, Polak JM. Tumor necrosis factor and inducible nitric oxide synthase in dilated cardiomyopathy. *Lancet* 1996;347:1151–1155.

29. Hattler BG, Gorcsan JIII, Shah N, Oddis CV, Billiar TR, Simmons RL, Finkel MS. A potential role for nitric oxide (NO) in myocardial stunning. *J Card Surg* 1994;9:425–429.

30. Hattler BG, Oddis CV, Zeevi A, Luss H, Shah N, Geller DA, Billiar TR, Simmons RL, Finkel MS. Regulation of constitutive nitric oxide synthase activity by the human heart. *Am J Cardiol* 1995;76:957–959.

31. Kanai AJ, Mesaros S, Finkel MS, Oddis CV, Strauss HC, Malinski T. Nitric oxide release measured directly with a porphyrinic microsensor reveals adrenergic control of constitutive nitric oxide synthase in cardiac myocytes. *Am J Physiol* 1997;273(42):C1371–C1377.

32. Kan H, Xie Z, Finkel MS. Norepinephrine stimulated MAP kinase activity enhances cytokine induced nitric oxide production by neonatal rat cardiac myocytes. *Am J Physiol* 1999;276:H47–H52.

33. Kan H, Xie Z, Finkel MS. TNF enhances NO production by neonatal rat cardiac myocytes through MAP kinase mediated activation of NF-κB. *Am J Physiol* 1999;277:H1646–H1646.

34. Liu S, Schreur KD. G protein-mediated suppression of L-type Ca^{2+} current by interleukin-1 beta in cultured rat ventricular myocytes. *Am J Physiol* 1995;268(2Pt1):C339–C349.

35. Mery PF, Pavoine C, Belhassen L, Pecker F, Fishmeister R. Nitric oxide regulates cardiac Ca^{2+} current. *J Biol Chem* 1993;268:26286–26295.

36. Oddis CV, Simmons RL, Hattler BG, Finkel MS. cAMP enhances inducible nitric oxide synthase mRNA stability in cardiac myocytes. *Am J Physiol* 1995;H38(6):2044–2050.

37. Pagani FD, Baker LS, Hsi C, Knox M, Fink MP, Visner MS. Left ventricular systolic and diastolic dysfunction after infusion of tumor necrosis factor-α in conscious dogs. *J Clin Invest* 1992;90:389–398.

38. Rozanski GJ, Witt RC. IL-1 inhibits beta-adrenergic control of cardiac calcium current: role of L-arginine/nitric oxide pathway. *Am J Phys* 1994;267(5Pt2):H1753–H1758.

39. Shinke T, Takaoka H, Takeuchi M, Hata K, Kawai H, Okubo H, Kijima Y, Murata T, Yokoyama M. Nitric oxide spares myocardial oxygen consumption through attenuation of contractile response to β-adrenergic stimulation in patients with idiopathic dilated cardiomyopathy. *Circulation* 2000;101:1925–1930.

40. Tatsumi T, Matoba S, Kawahara A, Keira N, Shiraishi J, Akashi K, Kobara M, Tanaka T, Katamura M, Nakagawa C, Ohta B, Shirayama T, Takeda K, Asayama J, Fliss H, Nakagawa M. Cytokine-induced nitric oxide production inhibits mitochondrial energy production and impairs contractile function in rat cardiac myocytes. *J Am Coll Cardiol* 2000;35:1338–1346.

41. Xu L, Eu JP, Meissner G, Stamler JS. Activation of the cardiac calcium release channel (ryanodine receptor) by poly-s-nitrosylation. *Science* 1998;27(9):234–236.

42. Katz AM, ed. *Physiology of the heart*, 2nd ed. New York: Raven Press, 1992.

43. Abramson JJ, Trimm JL, Weden L, Salama G. Heavy metals induce rapid calcium release from sarcoplasmic reticulum vesicles isolated from skeletal muscle. *Proc Natl Acad Sci USA* 1983;80:1526–1530.

44. Finkel MS, Oddis CV, Romeo RC, Salama G. Positive inotropic effect of acetylcysteine in the cardiomyopathic Syrian hamster. *J Card Pharm* 1993;21:29–34.
45. Kelly RA, Balligand JL, Smith TW. Nitric oxide and cardiac function. *Circ Res* 1996;79:363–380.
46. Bredt DS, Hwang PM, Glatt CE, Lowenstein C, Reed RR, Snyder SH. Cloned and expressed nitric oxide synthase structurally resembles cytochrome P-450 reductase. *Nature* 1991;351:714–718.
47. Ignarro LJ, Buga GM, Wood KS, Byrns RE, Chaudhuri G. Endothelium-derived relaxing factor produced and released from artery and vein is nitric oxide. *Proc Natl Acad Sci USA* 1987;84:9265–9269.
48. Janssens SP, Shimouchi A, Quertermous T, Bloch DB, Bloch KD. Cloning and expression of cDNA encoding human endothelium-derived relaxing factor/nitric oxide synthase. *J Biol Chem* 1992;267:14519–14522.
49. Lyons C, Orloff B, Cunningham J. Molecular cloning and functional expression of an inducible nitric oxide synthase from a murine macrophage cell line. *J Biol Chem* 1992;267:6370–6374.
50. Xie QW, Cho HJ, Calaycay J, Mumford RA, Swiderek KM, Lee TD, Ding A, Troso T, Nathan C. Cloning and characterization of inducible nitric oxide synthase from mouse macrophages. *Science* 1992;256:225–228.
51. Abbas AK, Lichtman AH, Pober JS. *Cellular and molecular immunology*. Philadelphia: W. B. Saunders Company, 1991:226–242.
52. Ognibene FP, Rosenberg SA, Lotze MT, Skibber J, Parker MM, Shelhamer JH, Parillo JE. Interleukin-2 administration causes reversible hemodynamic changes and left ventricular dysfunction similar to those seen in septic shock. *Chest* 1988;94:750–754.
53. Oddis CV, Finkel MS. Cytokines and nitric oxide synthase inhibitor as mediators of adrenergic refractoriness in cardiac myocytes. *Eur J Pharmacol* 1997;320:167–174.
54. Frering B, Philip I, Dehoux M, Rolland C, Langlois JM, Desmonts JM. Circulating cytokines in patients undergoing normothermic cardiopulmonary bypass. *J Thorac Cardiovasc Sur* 1994;108:636–641.
55. Steinberg JB, Kapelanski DP, Olson JD, Weiler JM. Cytokine and complement levels in patients undergoing cardiopulmonary bypass. *J Thorac Cardiovasc Surg* 1993;106:1008–1016.
56. Guillen I, Blanes M, Gomez-Lechon MJ, Castell JV. Cytokine signaling during myocardial infarction: sequential appearance of IL-1β and IL-6. *Am J Physiol* 1995;269 (*Regulatory Integrative Comp. Physiol 38*):R229–R235.
57. Ikeda U, Ohkawa F, Seino Y, Yamamotor K, Hidaka Y, Kasahara T, Kawai T, Shimada K. Serum interleukin 6 levels become elevated in acute myocardial infarction. *J Mol Cell Cardiol* 1992;24:579–584.
58. Ikeda U, Maeda Y, Kawahara Y, Yokoyama M, Shimada K. Angiotensin II augments cytokine-stimulated nitric oxide synthesis in rat cardiac myocytes. *Circulation* 1995;92:2683–2689.
59. Feldman MC, Gwarthmey JC, Phillips P, Schoen F, Morgan JP. Reversal of the force-frequency relationship in working myocardium from patients with end-stage heart failure. *J Appl Cardiol* 1988;3:273–283.

7. Experimental Heart Failure Models of Cytokine Overexpression

Charles F. McTiernan, PhD, Toshi Kadokami, MD, Yun You Li, PhD, and Arthur M. Feldman MD, PhD

The Cardiovascular Institute of the UPMC Health System, 200 Lothrop Street, S-572 Scaife Hall, Pittsburgh, PA 15215

Heart failure secondary to systolic dysfunction is a progressive cardiovascular disease that affects over 5 million people in the U.S. While the initial cause of heart failure in most patients is myocardial damage, the heart usually accommodates to the damage. However, over time, the heart remodels with the development of cardiac dilatation, cellular hypertrophy, cell slippage, diminished adrenergic responsiveness, apoptosis and extracellular matrix fibrosis and restructuring. Over the past decade, there has been a substantive increase in our knowledge of the pathobiology of the development of the heart failure phenotype. This increased knowledge has in part been attributable to advances in the sciences of cell and molecular biology and their application to studies of the failing human heart. However, our improved understanding of the molecular and cellular events leading to the development of heart failure and in particular the transition from compensated to de-compensated myocardial function can also be attributed to studies of new and novel animal models. Indeed, it is studies in animal models that have contributed seminal information regarding the fundamental role of the pro-inflammatory cytokines in the development of the heart failure phenotype. This Chapter will review in detail the observations from animal models that have supported the "Cytokine Hypothesis" of heart failure and will detail how animal models of cytokine over-expression have provided novel experimental platforms for evaluating the efficacy of anti-cytokine pharmacotherapy.

The first animal models to assess the role of cytokines in cardiovascular pathology were based on the hypothesis that the release of inflammatory mediators, including the pro-inflammatory cytokine TNFα, from activated white blood cells mediated the cardiovascular compromise that accompanies septic shock. In 1989, Natanson et al first recognized that the administration of either endotoxin or tumor necrosis factor to dogs effected changes in the cardiovascular profile that resembled those seen in human with septic shock [1]. Subsequent studies demonstrated that the intravenous infusion of a single dose of recombinant human TNFα (100 ug/kg) in canine resulted in a decrease in cardiac contractility, an increased in left ventricular dimension, and an increase in diastolic elastic stiffness [2–5]. The finding that these changes in cardiac morphology and function could only be appreciated six hours after the infusion and were persistent for up to 48 hours led investigators to hypothesize that second messengers and/or alterations in gene expression played a role in mediating the cardiotoxic effects of TNFα [6]. Furthermore, the recognition by Kapadia et al. in 1995 that adult mammalian myocardium could synthesize biologically active TNFα led to the recognition that cardiac production of TNFα could lead to depression of ventricular performance independent of systemic production or granulocyte activation. However, because these in vivo studies used relatively high doses of TNF for only short periods of time, the relevance of chronic TNF administration to the development of cardiac failure remained undefined.

In 1998, Bozkurt et al. administered TNFα to rats using osmotic infusion pumps implanted into the peritoneal space [7]. Systemic levels of biologically active TNFα were comparable to those reported in patients with heart failure (~80 to 100 U/ml) and resulted in a time-dependent depression in left ventricular function, cardiac myocyte shortening, and left ventricular dilatation. Myocardial histology by light microscopy was not altered by TNFα infusion and there was no evidence of interstitial inflammation or edema; however, there was a small but significant increase in myocyte size. By contrast, TNF exposure markedly affected the extracellular matrix as demonstrated by a marked decrease in collagen content and a disruption of the collagen weave that encapsulates the myocytes. However, apoptosis and TNFα-induced double-strand DNA breaks were not obvious. Thus, these studies strongly suggested that pathophysiologically rele-

Douglas L. Mann. THE ROLE OF INFLAMMATORY MEDIATORS IN THE FAILING HEART.
Copyright © 2001. Kluwer Academic Publishers. Boston. All rights reserved.

vant concentrations of TNFα could mimic at least in part the pathology seen in clinical heart failure.

As an alternative approach to assessing the role of pro-inflammatory cytokines in the development of heart failure we created lines of transgenic mice with constituitive over-expression of TNFα. This approach had several advantages: 1) we could assess the effects of TNF over longer periods of time; and 2) the effects of cardiac-restricted TNF expression could be measured. Initially, transgenic strains of mice (in the FVB background) were created by driving expression of the coding sequence of murine TNF-α with the murine alpha-myosin heavy chain promoter. To insure robust expression of the transgene, the 3'-untranslated region of TNF-α was replaced with that of the simian virus 40 T antigen—thus eliminating an AU-rich sequence found in the 3'-untranslated region of the TNFα gene that destabilizes the TNFα mRNA [8]. All transgenic mice (in the FVB strain) containing this construct (designated TNF.1) died shortly after birth and histologic examination of their hearts revealed a diffuse lymphohistiocytic myocarditis and interstitial edema. However, by creating a second transgene construct in which the destabilizing sequence in the 3' tail of the TNFα cDNA was re-inserted, we were able to establish a stable murine transgenic line (TNF1.6, also in the FVB strain) [9]. That the level of TNFα expression has a profound effect on

the development of the mouse phenotype was evidenced by comparing myocardial levels of TNFα in the murine strain with lethal myocarditis (7.5 nanograms/mg homogenate protein) and in the stable TNF1.6 strain (1.5 nanograms/mg homogenate protein). Interestingly, a construct nearly identical to our TNF1.1 transgene was used to generate a stable line of mice with heart failure and characteristics similar to the TNF1.6 line [10]. However these mice made in a different strain (C57BL/6JXJL/J), expressed far lower levels of immuno-detectable TNFα (2–11 picograms/mg protein).

The over-expression of TNFα resulted in the development of a dilated cardiomyopathy that recapitulated that seen in patients with heart failure. TNFα transgenic mice demonstrated: 1) left ventricular hypertrophy and dilatation; 2) augmentation of the "fetal gene program" including expression of atrial natriuretic factor mRNA and a shift in the myosin heavy chain isoform; 3) significantly blunted adrenergic responsiveness; and 4) a six-month mortality of approximately 23% (Fig. 1). Changes in the interstitium were obvious by routine light microscopy and included a mild, diffuse, lymphohistiocytic inflammatory infiltrate. There was also mild interstitial edema, an apparent increase in the production of matrix material, and focal interstitial fibrosis. Although apoptotic cell death was evident both by routine light microscopy and by

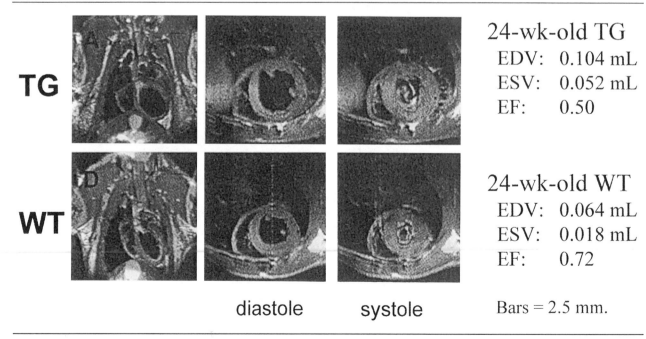

Fig. 1. *Representative Magnetic Resonance Images (MRI) from a 24 week old transgenic mouse (A, B, and C) and an age-matched wild type control (D, E, and F). Panels A and D illustrate coronal views of the mice; panels B and E, midventricular short axis views of the heart in end diastole; and panels C and F, midventricular short axis views of the heart in end systole [9].*

TUNEL assay ($\sim 0.3\%$ total nuclei were apoptotic), the predominant cell type undergoing apoptosis was CD45+ and actinin negative with very few actinin positive cells (0.04% total), presumed to be cardiomyocytes, scored as apoptotic. Consistent with the finding of increased apoptosis, over-expression of TNFα was associated with marked increase in the expression of a group of constitutively expressed death-domain related proteins including Fas, FADD, TRADD, and RIP [11]. In addition, expression of caspase-1 through -8 was also enhanced in the TNF1.6 mice as was that of pro-apoptotic members of the Bcl-2 family. However, TNFα over-expression strongly induced anti-apoptotic members of the Bcl-2 family, the anti-apoptotic A1, and activated NF-kB, a potent mediator of anti-apoptotic pathways. Thus, these results suggested that TNFα by itself is not sufficient to induce apoptosis in cardiac myocytes in vivo, which are perhaps protected by the activation of anti-apoptotic pathways, while pro-apoptotic mechanisms reveal their effects through increased apoptosis of the non-cardiomyocytes, infiltrating cells.

Autopsies performed on transgenic mice that died spontaneously demonstrated extreme enlargement of the heart, increased lung weight, and pleural effusions with or without ascites. In addition, a large number of mice had organized thrombi in the atria while interstitial fibrosis was relatively severe in some animals. While the autopsy analysis led us to presume that most of the animals died because of progressive congestive heart failure, miniaturized radiotelemetry devices were implanted on the backs of mice

with one lead secured on the right shoulder and the other lead near the cardiac apex [12] so as to assess the role of arrhythmias in the death of the TNF1.6 mice. Transgenic mice had substantially more ventricular and atrial ectopic beats than did the wild-type controls. However, these changes were most notable in the older transgenic mice in whom frequent premature ventricular and supraventricular complexes, progressive slowing of heart rate, and frequent runs of ventricular ectopy were common. In addition, a large portion of older transgenic animals (48 weeks) had atrial fibrillation. Thus, while death could be attributable to worsening heart failure in many of the TNFα transgenics, ventricular and atrial arrhythmias may also be a contributing factor, resembling the situation in human heart failure in which ventricular arrhythmias contribute to a significant mortality.

The TNF1.6 mice developed extensive fibrosis and extracellular matrix remodeling similar to that seen in patients with heart failure [13]. Remodeling during the development of heart failure appears to be regulated at least in part by the metalloproteinases, a family of functionally related enzymes that cleave matrix components, resulting in fibrillar collagen denaturation and degradation, and the synthesis of new fibrotic tissue (Fig. 2) [14–17]. Indeed, over-expression of MMP-1 leads to loss of cardiac interstitial collagen and the development of systolic and diastolic dysfunction [18]. In the TNF1.6 mice, progressive ventricular hypertrophy and dilatation were accompanied by a significant increase in MMP-2 and MMP-9 activity, an increase in

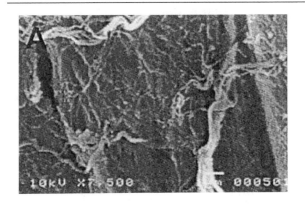
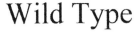

Wild Type

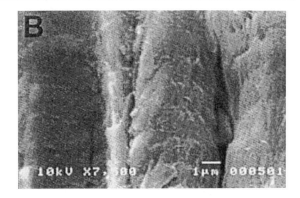

TNF1.6

Fig. 2. *Scanning electron micrographs from normal wild type mice (A) and transgenic mice (TNF1.6) with heart failure (B). While areas displaying loss of fine collagen fiber weave and struts are apparent in heart failure mice (B), other regions from the same heart may display significantly thickened and increased fibrillar collagen weave (not shown), suggesting a complex process of both collagen degradation and synthesis. Courtesy of F. Spinale, M.D., Ph.D.*

collagen synthesis, deposition, and denaturation, and a decrease in undenatured collagen [19]. These observations were not surprising as previous studies had demonstrated that the MMPs are increased in response to TNFα [20–23]. That these changes in the extracellular matrix were of physiologic importance was demonstrated by the finding that activation of the MMPs and matrix remodeling was associated with a marked reduction in diastolic function.

Another interesting feature of the TNF1.6 transgenic mice was a marked sex-related difference in survival: the 6-month survival rate of male and female TNF1.6 mice was 52% and 89% respectively (Fig. 3) [24]. In addition, TNF1.6 mice demonstrated sex-related differences in cardiac phenotype. Male TNF1.6 mice exhibited marked left ventricular dilatation and relatively thin walls, with reduced fractional shortening and marked blunting of isoproterenol responsiveness at 6 weeks of age. By contrast, left ventricular wall thickness but not chamber dimension was increased in female TNF1.6 mice, with diminished but persistent iosproterenol responsiveness. These findings could not be attributed to differences in heart rate, level of cytokine expression (including TNFα, IL-1B, TGF-B1, and MCP-1), or the amount of interstitial infiltrates. However, marked differences were observed between the levels of mRNA encoding both myocardial TNF receptors (TNFR1 and TNFR2). Indeed, the levels of TNFR1 mRNA were twice as high in male TNF1.6 mice while levels of TNFR2 mRNA were nearly fivefold higher. Interestingly, these elevations were also obvious in wild-type controls. The physiologic

significance of these increases in mRNA levels was demonstrated by the finding that the ability of TNFα to elicit the production of the TNFα-responsive second messenger molecule ceramide was significantly enhanced in male hearts relative to females.

Importantly, the differences in both TNFR mRNA levels and ceramide responsiveness could also be demonstrated in the hearts of wild type mice (FVB strain), but not in non-cardiac tissues of either TNF1.6 or wild type mice. This observation suggested that unique regulatory mechanisms within the heart were responsible for these gender-related differences in survival. In addition, recent studies have demonstrated that sex hormones may play a role in the cardio-protection afforded by female gender as exposure of male TNF1.6 mice to estrogen prior to, but not after, the development of puberty effected a marked improvement in survival [25]. However, it should be noted that in a recent study by Mann and colleagues (Mann et al, personal communication) they were unable to identify sex-related differences in survival in a TNFα over-expressing transgenic mice created using a construct in which the mRNA destabilizing region had been deleted [26]. These mice differed from the TNF1.6 mice in that levels of myocardial TNFα were substantially higher, TNF was expressed in the peripheral circulation as well as in the heart, and the background strain of the transgenic mice was different. Thus, while over-expression of TNF results in the development of marked cardiac pathology and signs of heart failure, the specific and unique phenotype of any transgenic animal is dependent on its unique genetic background. This finding is not without precedent as it is well-recognized that various strains of mice will respond quite differently when exposed to either a protein antigen or to a pathogenic virus [27]. Furthermore, the finding of gender-related differences in survival in the TNF1.6 mice is consistent with recent studies by Anversa and colleagues demonstrating that the female heart is protected, at least in part, from necrotic and apoptotic death signals [28] and recent clinical studies demonstrating improved survival in patients with heart failure [29].

Because the heart expresses TNFα in the presence of a variety of physiologic stresses, it is also possible to develop 'heart failure' models with cytokine over-expression by perturbing the normal physiology of the heart. Models of viral myocarditis show enhanced expression of proinflammatory cytokines (TNFα, IL-1β) in the acute phase of viral infection. However, elevated cardiac expression of IL-1β persists in the chronic, post-infection period in which a true heart failure may develop [30]. Thus prolonged

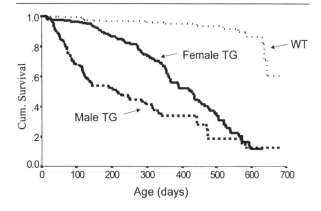

Fig. 3. *Survival function curve of TNF1.6 mice (n = 559) and wild-type littermates (n = 842). Female TNF1.6 mice (n = 401) survive significantly longer than male TNF1.6 mice (n = 158, p < 0.001). Mean survival time (limited to 360 days) for wild-type mice, female TNF1.6 mice, and male TNF1.6 mice was 346 ± 4, 286 ± 8, and 179 ± 12 days, respectively (mean ± SE) [24].*

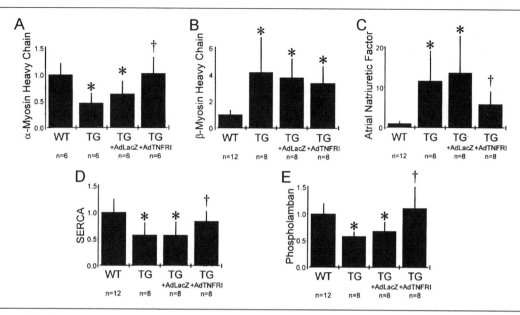

Fig. 4. *Expression of transcripts for cardiac specific genes are altered in TNF1.6 (TG) heart failure mice relative to wild type (WT) mice. Two weeks after treatment of TNF1.6 mice with an adenovirus expressing a human TNFRI-IgG fusion protein (AdTNFRI), expression of some transcripts were normalized, whereas treatment with a control adenovirus directing expression of E. coli β-galactosidase (AdLacZ) showed no effect [41].*

expression of IL-1β may participate in the development of heart failure and/or fibrosis after active viral myocarditis. As another example, the cardiac dilatation and failure seen in rat orthotopic cardiac allografts appears to be mediated at least in part by the expression of cardiac TNFα [31,32] and anti-TNF antibody therapy greatly enhanced cardiac allograft survival [33,34]. However, in these models, TNF serves to stimulate the activity and proliferation of immune active cells. Thus, the effects of TNF expression independent of its action as an inflammatory mediator in the transplant model is difficult to evaluate in immunocompetent rodents and in the presence of persistent antigen.

TNFα is also expressed in both the infarct and non-infarct zones in rodent models of myocardial infarction [35]. Expression of TNFα, IL-1β and IL-6 peaked at one week after infarction and decreased rapidly thereafter. However, the expression of these pro-inflammatory cytokines remained substantially elevated in the noninfarcted zone for up to 20 weeks after infarction. At one week post-infarction, the primary source of cytokine expression appears to be non-myocytes; however, the source of cytokine expression long-term after experimental infarction remains undefined [36]. Thus, cytokine expression may play an important role in the post-myocardial infarction remodeling process in the non-infarcted ventricular myocardium of rodents. However, a recent study demonstrates that endo-

genous TNFα protects the adult cardiac myocyte against ischemia-induced apoptosis as left ventricular infarct size after coronary ligation was substantially greater in TNFR1/TNFR2 deficient trangenic mice [37]. While the extent of necrosis did not differ, the frequency and extent of apoptosis was accelerated.

While rodents with experimentally-induced myocardial infarctions might provide another useful model for studying the biology of pro-inflammatory cytokines and their role in remodeling, it will be important to determine the time course of cytokine expression, relationships between cytokine expression and cellular biology, the post-myocardial infarction phenotype of the non-infarcted muscle, and the pathobiology of the non-infarct zone including extracellular matrix remodeling and fibrosis, apoptosis, and cellular function. The recent development of mouse infarct models will lead to important observations as experiments can be performed in transgenic mice harboring selective mutations in important cellular pathways.

A relatively straightforward means of creating a TNFα 'over-expression state' is to inject lipopolysaccharide (LPS) into the peritoneal cavity of rodents. While inexpensive and effective in increasing TNFα levels in both the heart and peripheral circulation, this strategy has important limitations as LPS activates the entire cytokine cascade including but not limited to IL-1B, IL-6, MCP-1, and a variety of chemokines. This generalized activation of pro-inflammatory cytokines appears to be independent of TNFα expression. For example, when LPS is administered to mice harboring a deletion of both the lymphotoxin α and TNFα genes, the absence of TNF does not confer long-term protection from lethality [38]. Similarly, anti-TNF therapy did not abrogate the expression of other pro-inflammatory cytokines in mice with LPS-induced endotoxemia [39]. Thus, administration of either LPS or endotoxin may not represent the in vivo cytokine milieu.

An important opportunity afforded by the development of heart failure models of cytokine over-expression is the ability to test the effectiveness of anti-cytokine therapies in vivo. Two anti-cytokine approaches have proven successful in both in vivo and in vitro experiments: soluble tumor necrosis factor receptors (sTNFR) and monoclonal anti-TNF antibodies. Both the soluble TNFR1 and TNFR2 receptors will neutralize bio-active TNF by competitively binding free TNF; however, the most robust neutralizing effects on a molar basis were obtained with a dimeric binding protein consisting of two molecules of the human soluble TNFR2 receptor linked by the Fc portion of the human immunoglobulin G1 molecule (IgG) [40]. These compounds effectively reversed the negative inotropic effects of TNF in cultured cardiac myocytes [40] and at least partially reversed the effects of continuous TNFα infusion in rats [7].

To better understand the long-term effects of anti-TNF therapy in vivo, we treated transgenic mice over-expressing TNFα with the chimeric human 55-kDa TNF soluble receptor (sTNFR:Fc). To effect prolonged exposure of transgenic mice to sTNFR:Fc, we expressed sTNFR:Fc using a replication-deficient recombinant adenovirus (AdTNFRI) [41]. A single intravenous injection of AdTNFR1 effected the production of a substantial amount of TNFRI in the plasma for as long as 6 weeks, largely due to uptake of virus and subsequent protein production by the liver. When injected into 6-week-old transgenic mice, AdTNFR1 blocked the myocardial expression of down-stream cytokines and chemokines including IL-1β and MCP-1, blocked the induction of intercellular adhesion molecule-1, and abrogated the development of interstitial infiltrates and myocarditis. In addition, treatment with AdTNFR1 effectively restored a more normal molecular phenotype as evidenced by normalization of the expression of sarcoplasmic reticulum Ca^{2+}-ATPase, phospholamban, and α-myosin heavy chain and effected normalization of the left ventricular end-systolic diameter. Interestingly, AdTNFR1 did not effect the TNFα-induced upregulation of β-MHC expression nor

did it fully suppress the enhanced expression of ANF. Consistent with the persistent up-regulation of β-MHC, AdTNFR1 did not influence TNFα-induced hypertrophy as measured either by gravitometric or echocardiographic indices. The ability to limit the progression of heart failure in animal models is not exclusive to treatment with sTNFR as similar salutary effects on disease progression were seen when TNF1.6 mice were treated with a monoclonal anti-TNFα antibody [42]. Thus, these studies, albeit in young animals, suggested the potential utility of anti-TNF therapies in patients with heart failure.

Anti-TNFα treatment with AdTNFR1 also attenuated the expression of both MMP-2 and MMP-9, prevented further collagen synthesis, deposition and denaturation in 12-week-old TNF1.6 mice [19]. Indeed, the activity of MMP-9 was abolished after 2 weeks of anti-TNFα therapy whereas MMP-2 activity was reduced to wild-type levels after 6 weeks of treatment. Furthermore, AdTNFR1 treatment prevented the increase in both total collagens and total soluble collagens that were found in the TNF1.6 mice and normalized the collagen phenotype. That these salutary changes in the components of the extracellular matrix had a physiologic effect was demonstrated by the fact that AdTNFR1 therapy was associated with a significant improvement in diastolic performance (Fig. 5). These results are similar to those seen after inhibition of MMP in mice after experimental myocardial infarction [43] and in swine with pacing-induced heart failure [44]. In both cases, MMP inhibition is associated with preservation of left ventricular size and function. However, the marked physiologic benefits seen with anti-cytokine therapy in 12-week-old transgenic mice was not obvious in 48-week-old mice as both left ventricular end-diastolic dimension and fractional shortening remained virtually unchanged after treatment (Table 1). Consistent with these observations, treatment with a metalloproteinase antagonist effectively attenuated maladaptive cardiac remodeling and improved survival in young but not old TNF1.6 mice [45].

While studies in animal models strongly support the hypothesis that anti-TNF therapy can be beneficial in patients with heart failure, it appears that the therapeutic window might be narrow and limited to animals in whom significant extracellular matrix remodeling has not yet occurred. Cytokines mediated changes in the extracellular matrix include a shift in collagen phenotype and a reduction in the number of thick collagen fibers connecting adjoining muscle fiber bundles [46]. These changes result in the loss of the supportive scaffolding of the heart which in turn leads to cell slippage and ventricular dilation. The resulting intracellular spaces are 'filled-in' by

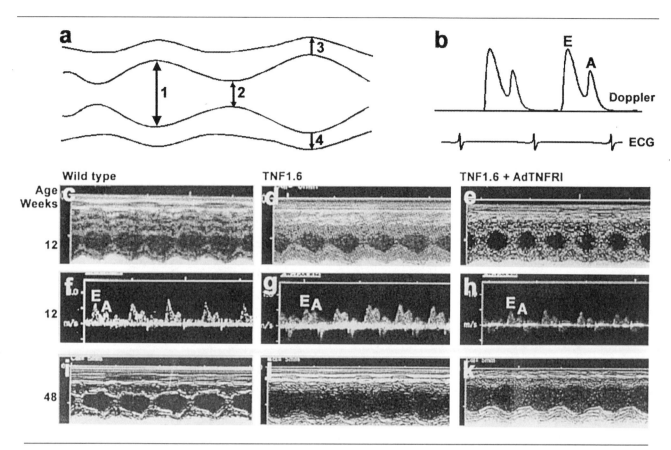

Fig. 5.. *Echocardiographic measurement of the geometry and function of the mouse heart. LV dimensions were calculated from measurements of end-diastolic diameter (**1**), end-systolic diameter (**2**), anterior wall (**3**), and posterior wall (**4**), and E/A wave ratio was calculated as shown in schematic M-mode (**a**) and Doppler (**b**) echocardiographic tracings. Ventricular hypertrophy in 12 week old TNF1.6 mice (**d**), ventricular dilation in 48 week old TNF1.6 mice (**j**) as compared to respective wild type mice (**c, i**). AdTNFRI treatment had no effect on ventricular hypertrophy or dilation (**e, k**), but the reduced E/A ratio in 12-week-old TNF1.6 mice (**g**) was prevented by the treatment (**h**) [19].*

reparative fibrosis; however, the replacement collagen is poorly cross-linked and therefore increases the overall stiffness of the heart. Thus, while anti-cytokine therapy might attenuate or even abrogate this process of remodeling early in the development of heart failure, studies in animal models of TNFα over-expression suggest that anti-TNF therapy may be unable to restore the original

Table 1. *Measurements of mouse myocardial structure and function*

Age (Weeks)	Measurement	Wild type (Mean ± SD, n = 4)	TNF1.6 (Mean ± SD, n = 6)	TNF1.6 + AdTNFRI (Mean ± SD, n = 6)
12	VW/BW	3.92 ± 0.3	5.03 ± 0.41*	5.19 ± 0.39*
	LVED	3.72 ± 0.26	4.05 ± 0.19	3.8 ± 0.14
	FS (%)	37.11 ± 2.41	35.64 ± 3.00	38.97 ± 2.77
	FS (%) + Iso	59.53 ± 4.68‡	52.27 ± 15.19‡	54.25 ± 7.92‡
	E/A ratio	1.71 ± 0.30	1.26 ± 0.16*	1.58 ± 0.27§
48	VW/BW	3.49 ± 0.12	4.86 ± 0.22*	4.62 ± 0.57*
	LVED	3.79 ± 0.17	4.63 ± 0.59*	4.27 ± 0.31*
	FS (%)	40.18 ± 7.81	27.1 ± 6.50*	28.91 ± 2.53*
	FS (%) + Iso	65.7 ± 15.7‡	29.82 ± 2.35‡	37.55 ± 3.78‡

VW, ventricular weight (mg); BW, body weight (g); LVED, left ventricular end diastolic diameter (mm); FS, fractional shortening; Iso, isoproterenol. *: $P < 0.05$ vs wild type; ‡: $P < 0.01$ vs Iso unchallenged; ‡: $P < 0.05$ vs Iso challenged TNF1.6 + AdTNFRI; §: $P < 0.05$ vs TNF1.6

complex three-dimensional architecture that is critical for effective pump performance.

Although investigations to date have characterized the phenotype of heart failure models of cytokine over-expression, these models provide a unique opportunity to further understand cardiac biology. For example, recent studies have demonstrated that TNFα can modify the phenotype of the cardiac vasculature including induction of neointimal hyperplasia [47] and promotion of osteoblastic differentiation of vascular cells [48]. However, studies to date have not evaluated the coronary vasculature in TNFα over-expressing mice. The use of mouse models of TNFα over-expression also allows for cross-breeding with transgenic mice harboring mutations in selective receptors or down-stream effector proteins allowing investigators the opportunity to identify those cellular pathways that are critical for the development of the heart failure phenotype. Such studies might also help to identify novel therapeutic targets that are cardiac specific.

Because the development of heart failure in animal models over-expressing TNFα has been thoroughly characterized and is highly consistent within each transgenic strain, new technologies including differential display and micro-chip arrays can be utilized to identify unique genes that are differentially expressed during the development of heart failure. Finally, experimental heart failure models of cytokine over-expression can also be used to screen new anti-cytokine therapeutic agents. Although effective in ameliorating the bio-activity of TNF in vivo, both recombinant soluble TNF receptors and partially humanized monoclonal antibodies have therapeutic limitations including high cost, need for subcutaneous or intravenous administration, generalized inhibition of TNFα, and limited usefulness due to inherent immunogenicity (in the case of monoclonal antibodies). Thus, there will be a need for new and cardiac specific anti-TNF agents.

In summary, pro-inflammatory cytokines play an important role in the development of the heart failure phenotype. Our understanding of the role of cytokines has been greatly facilitated by the development of experimental heart failure models of cytokine over-expression. These models have included activation of endogenous TNFα expression by endotoxin or LPS, chronic infusion of recombinant TNFα using surgically implanted mini-pumps, and transgenic over-expression of TNFα in mice. Taken together, the results of these studies clearly demonstrate a role for TNFα in the development of heart failure. Indeed, cardiac-restricted over-expression of TNFα effects the development of a cardiac phenotype that virtually recapitulates that seen in humans with this disease. In addition, the devel-

opment of heart failure models over-expressing TNFα have led to identification of cellular regulatory pathways that appear to be critical for expression of the phenotype. Importantly, these animal models have also provided an investigational platform with which to assess the efficacy of anti-cytokine or anti-metalloproteinase pharmacotherapeutics—studies that have provided important clues as to the optimal therapeutic window for these agents. Finally, experimental heart failure models of cytokine over-expression should also provide important tools with which to identify and define new and novel therapeutic targets. While these novel models have been extensively characterized, a large amount of additional information is likely to be obtained from further studies and these studies will hopefully lead to improved outcomes for patients with heart failure.

References

1. Natanson C, Eichenholz PW, Danner RL, Eichacker W, Hoffman D, Kuo SM, Banks TJ, MacViottie TJ, Parrillo JE. Endotoxin and tumor necrosis factor challenges in dogs simulate the cardiovascular profile of human septic shock. *J Exp Med* 1989;169:823–832.

2. McMurray JJ, Abdullah I, Dargie HJ, Shapiro D. Increased concentrations of tumour necrosis factor in 'cachectic' patients with severe chronic heart failure. *Br Heart J* 1991;66:356–358.

3. Eichenholz PW, Eichacker PQ, Hoffman WD, Banks SM, Parrillo JEDR, Natanson C. Tumor necrosis factor challenges in canines: patterns of cardiovascular dysfunction. *Am J Physiol* 1992;263:H668–H675.

4. Walley KR, Hebert PC, Wakai Y, Wilcox PG, Road JD, Cooper DJ. Decrease in left ventricular contractility after tumor necrosis factor-α infusion in dogs. *J Appl Physiol* 1994;76:1060–1067.

5. Murray DR, Freeman GL. Tumor necrosis factor-α induces a biphasic effect on myocardial contractility in conscious dogs. *Circ Res* 1996;78:154–160.

6. Pagani FD, Baker LS, Hsi C, Knox M, Fink MP, Visner MS. Left ventricular systolic and diastolic dysfunction after infusion of tumor necrosis factor-α in conscious dogs. *J Clin Invest* 1992;90:389–398.

7. Bozkurt B, Kribbs SB, Clubb FJ, Jr., Michael LH, Didenko VV, Hornsby PJ, Seta Y, Oral H, Spinale FG, Mann DL. Pathophysiologically relevant concentrations of tumor necrosis factor-alpha promote progressive left ventricular dysfunction and remodeling in rats. *Circulation* 1998;97:1382–1391.

8. Kubota T, McTiernan CF, Frye CS, Demetris AJ, Feldman AM. Cardiac-Specific Overexpression of tumor necrosis factor-Alpha Causes lethal myocarditis in transgenic mice. *Journal of Cardiac Failure* 1997;3:117–124.

9. Kubota T, McTiernan CF, Frye CS, Slawson SE, Koretsky AP, Demetris AJ, Feldman AM. Dilated cardiomyopathy in transgenic mice with cardiac-specific overexpression of tumor necrosis factor-alpha. *Circ Res* 1997;81:627–635.

10. Bryant D, Becker L, Richardson J, Shelton J, Franco F, Peschock R, Thompson M, Giroir B. Cardiac failure in transgenic mice with myocardial expression of tumor necrosis factor-α. *Circulation* 1998;97:1375–1381.
11. Kubota T, Miyagishima M, Bounoutas GS, Kadokami T, Watkins SC, McTiernan CF, Feldman AM. Overexpression of tumor necrosis factor-α activates both anti- and pro-apoptotic pathways in the myocardium. *J Mol Cell Cardiol* 2000;in press
12. Shusterman V, Usiene I, Aysin B, Feldman AM, London B. Slow rhythm destabilization precedes initiation of ventricular arrhythmias in a TNF-? Mouse model of congestive heart failure. *NASPE* in press: (Abstract)
13. Weber KT. Cardiac interstitium in health and disease: The Fibrillar Collagen Network. *J Am Coll Cardiol* 1989;13:1637–1652.
14. Dollery CM, McEwan JR, Henney AM. Matrix metalloproteinases and cardiovascular disease. *Circulation Research* 1995;77:863–868.
15. Spinale FG, Tomita M, Thomas CV, Walker JD, Mukherjee R, Hebbar L. Time-dependent changes in matrix metalloproteinase activity and selective upregulation in LV myocardium from patients with end-stage dilated cardiomyopathy. *Circulation Research* 1998;82:482–495.
16. Li YY, McTiernan CF, Feldman AM. Interplay of matrix metalloproteinases, tissue inhibitors of metalloproteinases and their regulators in cardiac matrix remodeling. *Cardiovascular Research* 2000;46:214–224.
17. Maquart FX, Pickart L, Laurent M, Gillery P, Monboisse JC, Borel JP. Stimulation of collagen synthesis in fibroblast cultures by the tripeptide-copper complex glycl-L-histidyl-L-lysine-Cu2 +. *FEBS Lett* 1988;238:343–346.
18. Kim HE, Dalal SS, Young E, Legato MJ, Weisfeldt ML, D'Armiento J. Disruption of the myocardial extracellular matrix leads to cardiac dysfunction. *J Clin Invest* 2000;106:857–866.
19. Li YY, Feng Q, Kadokami T, McTiernan CF, Watkins SC, Feldman AM. Myocardial extracellular matrix remodeling in transgenic mice overexpressing tumor necrosis factor-α can be modulated by anti-tumor necrosis factor-α therapy. *Proc Natl Acad Sci USA* 2000;97:12746–12751.
20. Li YY, McTiernan CF, Feldman AM. Proinflammatory cytokines regulate tissue inhibitors of metalloproteinases and disintegrin metalloproteinase in cardiac cells. *Cardiovascular Research* 1999;42:162–172.
21. Galis ZS, Muszynski M, Sukhova GK, Simon-Morrissey E, Libby P. Enhanced expression of vascular matrix metalloproteinases induced in vitro by cytokines and in regions of human atherosclerotic lesions. *Ann NY Acad Sci* 1995;748:501–507.
22. Lefebvre V, Peeters-Joris C, Vaees G. Production of gelatin-degrading matrix metalloproteinases ('type IV collagenases') and inhibitors by articular chondrocytes during their dedifferentiation by serial subcultures and under stimulation by interleukin-1 and tumor necrosis factor alpha. *Biochim Biophys Acta* 1991;1094:8–18.
23. Lee E, Vaughan DE, Parikh S, Grodzinsky AJ, Libby P, Lark MW, Lee RT. Regulation of matrix metallopro-

teinases and plasminogen activator inhibitor-1 synthesis by plasminogen in cultured human vascular smooth muscle cells. *Circ Res* 1996;78:44–49.
24. Kadokami T, McTiernan CF, Frye CS, Feldman AM. Sex-related survival differences in murine cardiomyopathy are associated with differences in TNF-receptor expression. *J Clin Invest* 2000;106:589–597.
25. Kadokami T, McTiernan CF, Kubota T, Feldman AM. Long term estradiol treatment improves survival in male mice with heart failure induced by cardiac specific TNF-expression. *Circulation* 102:II–72 (Abstract)
26. Li X, Moody MR, Engel D, Walker S, Clubb FJ, Jr., Sivasubramanian N, Mann DL, Reid MB. Cardiac-specific overexpression of tumor necrosis factor-α causes oxidative stress and contractile dysfunction in mouse diaphragm. *Circulation* 2000;102:1690–1696.
27. Feldman AM, McNamara DM. Medical Progress: Myocarditis. *N Eng J Med* 2000;343:1388–1398.
28. Guerra S, Len A, Wang X, Finato N, DiLoreto C, Beltrami CA, Kajstura J, Anversa P. Myoctye death in the failing human heart is gender dependent. *Circ Res* 1999;85:856–866.
29. Adams KF, Dunlap S, Sueta CA, Clarke SW, Patterson JH, Blauwet MB, Jensen LR, Tomasko L, Koch GG. Relation between gender, etiology and survival in patients with symptomatic heart failure. *J Am Coll Cardiol* 1996;28:1781–1788.
30. Shioi T, Matsumori A, Sasayama S. Persistent expression of cytokine in the chronic stage of viral myocarditis in mice. *Circulation* 1996;94:2930–2937.
31. Lowry RP, Blais D. Tumor necrosis factor-alpha in rejecting rat cardiac allografts. *Transplant Proc* 1988;20:245–247.
32. Maury CPJ, Teppo AM. Raised serum levels of cachectin/tumor necrosis factor in renal allograft rejection. *J Exp Med* 1987;166:1132–1137.
33. Bolling SF, Kunkel SL, Lin H. Prolongation of cardiac allograft survival in rats by anti-TNF and cyclosporine combination therapy. *Transplantation* 1992;53:283–286.
34. Lin H, Chensue SW, Strieter RM, Remick DG, Gallagher KP, Bolling, SF, Kunkel SL. Antibodies against tumor necrosis factor prolong cardiac allograft survival in the rat. *Journal of Heart & Lung Transplantation* 1992;11:330–335.
35. Ono K, Matsumori A, Shioi T, Furukawa Y, Sasayama S. Cytokine gene expression after myocardial infarction in rat hearts: possible implication in left ventricular remodeling. *Circulation* 1998;98:149–156.
36. Yue P. Massie BM, Simpson PC, Long CS. Cytokine expression increases in nonmyocytes from rats with postinfarction heart failure. *American Journal of Physiology* 1998;275:H250–H258.
37. Kurrelmeyer KM, Michael LH, Baumgarten G, Taffett GE, Peschon JJ, Sivasubramanian N, Entman ML, Mann DL. Endogenous tumor necrosis factor protects the adult cardiac myocyte against ischemic-induced apoptosis in a murine model of acute myocardial infarction. *Proc Natl Acad Sci USA* 2000;97:5456–5461.
38. Amiot F, Fitting C, Tracey KJ, Cavaillon JM, Dautry F. Lipopolysaccharide-induced cytokine cascade and lethality in LTα/TNFα-deficient mice. *Mol Med* 1997;3:864–875.

39. Kadokami T, Kubota T, Bounoutas GS, McTiernan CF, Feldman AM. Soluble tumor necrosis factor receptor differentially regulates cardiac cytokine gene expression in mice with lipopolysaccharide-induced endotoxemia. *Circulation* 1999;100:I–16 (Abstract)

40. Kapadia S, Torre-Amione G, Yokoyama T, Mann DL. Soluble TNF binding proteins modulate the negative inotropic properties of TNF-alpha in vitro. *American Journal of Physiology* 1995;268:H517–25.

41. Kubota T, Bounoutas GS, Miyagishima M, Kadokami T, Sanders VJ, Bruton C, Robbins PD, McTiernan CF, Feldman AM. Soluble tumor necrosis factor receptor abrogates myocardial inflammation but not hypertrophy in cytokine-induced cardiomyopathy. *Circulation* 2000;101:2518–2525.

42. McTiernan CF, Kadokami T, Lemster BH, Frye CS, Wagner CL, Feldman AM. Anti-TNF antibody limits progression of heart failure in a murine transgenic model. *Circulation* 2000;102:II–265 (Abstract)

43. Rohde LE, Ducharme A, Arroyo LH, et al. Matrix metalloproteinase inhibition attenuates early left ventricular enlargement after experimental myocardial infarction in mice. *Circulation* 1999;99:3063–3070.

44. Spinale FG, Coker ML, Krombach SR, Mukherjee R, Hallak H, Houck WV, Clair MJ, Kribbs SB, Johnson LL, Peterson JT, Zile MR. Matrix metalloproteinase inhibition during the development of congestive heart failure. Effects on left ventricular dimensions and function. *Circ Res* 1999;85:364–376.

45. Li YY, Feng YQ, Kadokami T, McTiernan CF, Feldman AM. Modulation of matrix metalloproteinase activities remodels myocardial extracellular matrix in TNFα transgenic mice. *Circulation* 1999; 100:I–752 (Abstract)

46. Gunja-Smith Z, Morales AR, Romanelli R, Woessner JF. Remodeling of human myocardial collagen in idiopathic dilated cardiomyopathy: role of metalloproteinases and pyridinoline cross links. *American Journal of Physiology* 1996;148:1639–1648.

47. Rectenwald JE, Moldawer LL, Huber TS, Seeger JM, Ozaki CK. Direct evidence for cytokine involvement in neointimal hyperplasia. *Circulation* 2000;102:1697–1702.

48. Tinut Y, Patel J, Parhami F, Demer LL. Tumor necrosis factor-α promotes in vitro calcification of vascular cells via the cAMP pathway. *Circulation* 2000;102:2636–2642.

8. Immunomodulation of Cytokines in Experimental Models of Heart Failure

Akira Matsumori, MD, PhD and
Shigetake Sasayama, MD, PhD
Department of Cardiovascular Medicine, Kyoto University,
Graduate School of Medicine

Introduction

Congestive heart failure (CHF) may be produced by a variety of disorders, including dilated cardiomyopathy, hypertensive heart disease, and ischemic heart disease. We have developed experimental models of these diseases. In a murine model of myocarditis, inflammatory cytokines were induced rapidly in the myocardium, and remained expressed during the chronic stage, when the heart had developed the typical characteristics of dilated cardiomyopathy. In the pressure-overloaded ventricle, the myocardium developed adaptive hypertrophy before its transition to heart failure, a process in which cytokines appeared to play a significant role by accelerating myocyte growth and down-modulating cardiac function. In the ischemic heart, the non-ischemic myocardium developed hypertrophy associated with progression of scarring in the ischemic area. This remodeling process initially represents an important compensatory mechanism to preserve ventricular function, though later leads to the development of heart failure. During this phase of healing from acute ischemia, inflammatory cytokines were persistently upregulated in the non-ischemic myocardium. Thus, we hypothesized that some aspects of heart failure may be mediated by reversible alterations of cardiac function and structural changes in the ventricle induced by cytokines. In the respect, several drugs used routinely in clinical practice have been proved to modulate the production of cytokines, suggesting that immunomodulating or anticytokine therapy may represent a new approach to the management of heart failure [1].

There is growing evidence that immunologic responses mediated by cytokines play an important pathogenic role in the development of heart failure (Fig. 1). Several clinical studies have shown that patients with CHF express excessive levels of cytokines in the blood [2–6]. This review discusses the process of immunomodulation in experimental models of heart failure.

Cytokines in experimental models of heart failure due to myocarditis and cardiomyopathy

We have developed murine models of viral myocarditis induced by the encephalomyocarditis virus (EMCV), associated with a high incidence of severe myocarditis, CHF and dilated cardiomyopathy. From these models we have observed the natural history and pathogenesis of viral myocarditis, and tested new diagnostic methods, as well as therapeutic and preventive interventions [7,8]. During the first 7 days, the virus replicates in the myocardium and directly causes myocytolysis. Histopathological examination of the myocardium revealed that the cellular infiltration and myocardial necrosis developed during this period. Then, CHF became apparent from 7 to 10 days postinfection onwards, by which time most of the culturable virus has been eliminated, though the viral genome can be detected by PCR [9]. To study the role of TNF-α in this model, we measured plasma TNF-α levels by enzyme-linked immunosorbent assay (ELISA), and examined the effects of recombinant human TNF-α [10] and of anti-murine TNF-α monoclonal antibody (mAb) *in vivo* [11]. Plasma TNF-α concentration was increased in the blood of infected mice, 3–7 days after virus inoculation. The myocardial viral content was higher in the TNF-α-treated group than in the control group. Histopathological analysis revealed that myocardial necrosis and cellular infiltration were more prominent in the TNF-α group than in the control group. Anti-TNF-α mAb improved survival and myocardial lesions when treatment was initiated 1 day before virus inoculation. However, it had no therapeutic effect when administered on the day inoculation or the next day. TNF-α may play an important role in the very early stages of the immune response, and anti-TNF-α mAb may block the early pathway of acute viral myocarditis [11].

Douglas L. Mann. *THE ROLE OF INFLAMMATORY MEDIATORS IN THE FAILING HEART.*
Copyright © 2001. Kluwer Academic Publishers. Boston. All rights reserved.

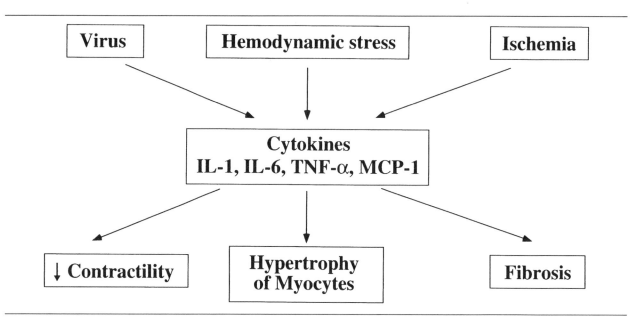

Fig. 1.   *Cytokines and the heart. Viral infection, hemodynamic stress and ischemia induce the production of cytokines, which may depress myocardial contractility, induce hypertrophy of myocytes, and fibrosis.*

We also studied the expression of cytokine messenger RNA (mRNA) in our model [12]. IL-1β and TNF-α mRNAs were induced 3 days after inoculation, when few cellular infiltrates were observed, suggesting that, at that stage, these cytokines were produced by intrinsic cells in the heart tissue. Immunohistochemical analysis revealed that endothelial cells and interstitial macrophages were positive for IL-1β and TNF-α immunoreactivity 3 days after inoculation. The expression of these cytokines is likely to influence the induction of the local inflammatory process [13]. Interferon (IFN)-γ mRNA appeared 3 days, and IL-2 mRNA 7 days after inoculation. T cell infiltration within the heart peaked at days 7 to 14 after inoculation in this model. A temporal correlation between cellular infiltration and IL-2 and IFN-γ mRNA production suggests that infiltrating cells, rather than resident heart cells, account for the appearance of IFN-γ and IL-2 mRNA in the heart. IFN-γ and IL-2 proteins are likely to be produced, since the production of IFN-γ and IL-2 is regulated mainly at the transcriptional level. One of the most important findings of our study was the persistent expression of IFN-γ, IL-1β, IL-2 and TNF-α for as long as 80 days after virus inoculation. IL-2, which is produced exclusively by T lymphocytes, is likely to originate from infiltrating mononuclear cells, which are occasionally seen 80 days after inoculation. The presence of IL-2 mRNA suggests that T-cells, activated in a major histocompatibility complex (MHC)-dependent manner, are

present in the heart tissue in the chronic stage. The temporal expression of IL-2 and IFN-γ mRNA in the chronic phases was correlated with that of the EMCV genome RNA. This suggests that the expression of IL-2 and IFN-γ is triggered by persistent viral infection in this model, although autoimmune mechanisms should also be considered, since, in a rat model, focal accumulation of mononuclear cells was preceded by myosin-induced autoimmune myocarditis. In our study, IL-1β gene expression in the chronic stage was relatively high compared with other cytokines, and was positively correlated with the heart weight/body weight ratio and with the extent of fibrotic lesions, suggesting a possible role of IL-1β in the pathogenesis of cardiomyopathic changes in this model. IFN-γ, IL-2 and TNF-α gene expressions in the chronic stage were not significantly correlated with heart weight/body weight ratio or extent of fibrosis.

Cytokines in an experimental model of hypertensive heart failure

The left ventricle responds to an excessive mechanical load by dilatation and myocardial hypertrophy. Initially, these changes represent important compensatory mechanisms regulating chamber wall stress and maintaining a relatively normal pumping function. However, heart failure may ensue as a direct consequence of the finite ability, and ultimate failure, of this compensatory remodeling. We have recently developed an experimental model which allows a close evaluation of the sequence of events occurring during the transition from adaptive left ventricular hypertrophy to cardiac failure [14]. Dahl salt-sensitive rats fed with a high-salt diet rapidly developed typical left ventricular hypertrophy, and severe impairment of myocardial function with chamber dilation. In this model, an increased expression of IL-1β was observed in the hypertrophied heart, which was further increased with the development of CHF [15]. Immunohistochemical studies revealed that IL-1β protein was located in endothelial cells of the arterioles and in infiltrating macrophages within the hypertrophied myocardium. The amount of IL-1β mRNA correlated with the ventricular mass. The expression of monocyte chemoattractant protein-1/monocyte chemotactic and activating factor (MCP-1), a potent chemotactic factor for macrophages, was also increased, along with an increased number of macrophages in the interstitium. In fact, it has been suggested that macrophages activated by chemokines are important cellular sources of increased levels of circulating proinflammatory cytokines.

High circulating levels of chemokines have been found in patients with heart failure [16,17], as well as patients with acute myocardial infarction [18], and importance of chemokines in cardiovascular diseases has been reported [19], When cyclic mechanical stretch was applied to the endothelial cells of human umbilical veins cultured on flexible silicone membranes, concentrations of MCP-1 in the culture medium were significantly increased [20]. Northern blot analysis indicated that mRNA levels of MCP-1 were upregulated by cyclic stretch. Analysis with specific enzyme inhibitors showed that phospholipase C, protein kinase C and tyrosin kinase were also involved in this induction of chemokine [20]. The sum of these observations suggests that mechanical stretch induces gene expression of chemotactic factors for macrophages. Recruited macrophages are the main source of production of cytokines, notably IL-1β (Fig. 2). A continuous infusion of TNF-α into the peritoneal cavity of rats has been shown to cause a time-dependent depression of left ventricular function together with left ventricular dilation, suggesting that TNF-α promotes remodeling of the failing heart [21]. However, in our model, IL-1β appeared to play a major role. The transition of compensated hypertrophy to heart failure may be the result of a combination of several factors, structure and function of the myocytes being modulated not only by loading conditions, but also by systemic or local neurohumoral processes.

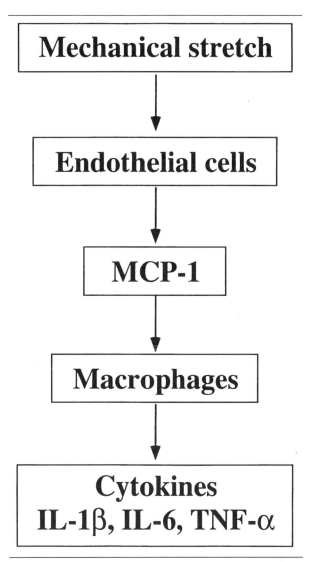

Fig. 2. *Hemodynamic stress and cytokines. Mechanical stretch induces expression of MCP-1 in endothelial cells, macrophages are recruited and activated by MCP-1, and these macrophages may produce cytokines.*

Cytokines in experimental model of heart failure due to myocardial infarction

During acute coronary occlusion, systolic shortening of the ischemic myocardium is rapidly replaced by a paradoxical systolic expansion with elongation of segment length. In the chronic stage, the scarring of the infarcted area proceeds with only minimal restoration of function. In the non-infarcted area, there is a progressive increase in end-diastolic length and extent of shortening, as is observed in conditions of chronic volume overload. This remodeling process initially represents an important compensatory mechanism for the preservation of ventricular pump function, though it may later lead to the development of CHF.

In a rat model of myocardial infarction, progressive dilation of the left ventricular cavity with impaired systolic shortening was imaged by transthoracic echocardiography [22]. In this experimental model, gene expression of TNF-α, IL-1β and IL-6 rose sharply in the infarcted region at 1 week after coronary occlusion, and decreased gradually thereafter to return to baseline values at 20 weeks. In contrast, in the noninfarcted region, upregulation of the expression of these cytokines was moderate at 1 week, but remained significantly increased throughout the study period. Concentrations of these cytokines in the noninfarcted region correlated with left ventricular enddiastolic diameter measured at 8 and 20 weeks after infarction. Among them, IL-1β expression was most prominent, and its concentration correlated well with collagen deposition in the noninfarcted myocardium in chronic stages [22]. We have recently reported that MCP-1 is also induced by myocardial ischemia/reperfusion, that neutralization of MCP-1 significantly reduces infarct size [23], and that neutralization of MCP-1 before, and immediately after arterial injury may be effective in preventing restenosis after angioplasty [24].

Immunomodulation of cytokines in experimental models of heart failure

Phospodiesterase inhibitors
Several proinflammatory cytokines are known to cause myocardial contractile dysfunction, with negative inotropic effects thought to be mediated by nitric oxide [25,26]. We have recently studied the effects of the PDE III inhibitors amrinone, pimobendan and vesnarinone, and have observed their different modulations of the production of these cytokines [27]. We have also studied the effects of amrinone, pimobendan, vesnarinone, and of the cell-permeable cyclic nucleotide analogue, 8-bromo adenosine 3'5'-cyclic monophosphate (8 Br-cAMP), on the induction of nitric oxide synthase by LPS in J774A.1 macrophages *in vitro*. Although the 3 inotropic agents inhibited nitrite accumulation, the degree of inhibition was variable, pimobendan being the most potent inhibitor and amrinone the least. 8 Br-cAMP increased nitrite production in high concentrations, suggesting that the inhibitory effects of the inotropic agents were not due to an increase in cAMP [28]. Thus, the variable inhibition of inducible nitric oxide synthase by inotropic agents suggested different effects of these drugs in patients with CHF. In our murine model of heart failure due to viral myocarditis, pimoben-

dan improved survival, attenuated inflammatory lesions, and decreased production of intracardiac IL-1β, IL-6 and TNF-α and nitric oxide [29]. However, the inhibitory mechanism of pimobendan on these mediators was not clarified.

In a recent study from our laboratory, pimobendan, but not the other PDE III inhibitors, inhibited activation of NF-κB. Like forskolin, NKH477 directly activates the catalytic unit of adenylate cyclase and increases cAMP. Since NKH did not suppress the activation of NF-κB either, inhibition of NF-κB activation by pimobendan was apparently not attributable to an increase in cAMP. The mechanism by which pimobendan inhibits NF-κB remains unclear.

The importance of intracellular free calcium in the regulation of cytokine expression has been established in human monocytes, and changes in calcium levels have been found to modulate the phosphorylation of IκB, which regulates the activation of NF-κB [30]. Since pimobendan possesses calcium-sensitizing properties, it may inhibit the activation of NF-κB by modulating these signal transduction pathways. Activation of NF-κB is critical for the expression of proinflammatory cytokines such as IL-1β, IL-6 and TNF-α, and inducible nitric oxide synthase, and plays an important role in the pathogenesis of inflammation and immunological diseases [31,32] Thus, the inhibitory effect of pimobendan on the production of proinflammatory cytokines and nitric oxide is explained by its inhibitory effect on the activation of NF-κB. The effect of pimobendan in heart failure may also be partially explained by this effect.

Digitalis
Digitalis has been a controversial drug since its introduction over 200 years ago. Although its efficacy in patients with CHF and atrial fibrillation is clear, its value in patients with CHF and sinus rhythm has often been questioned. The recently published results of the multicenter trial by the Digitalis Investigation Group indicate that, in a large population of patients with CHF, long-term treatment with digoxin had no significant effect on overall mortality, though it reduced the overall rate of hospital admissions and that for worsening heart failure. In another study, digoxin had an adverse effect on ventricular remodeling after myocardial infarction, despite an increase in ejection fraction. This finding has been reported before, though its clinical relevance is unclear. The growing awareness of neurohumoral activation as a contributing factor in the progression of chronic heart failure has redirected the attention of investigators toward the modulating effects of digoxin on

neurohumoral and autonomic states. We found recently that the cardiac glycoside ouabain induces the production of IL-1β, IL-6, and TNF-α in human peripheral blood mononuclear cells (PBMC) [33]. Ouabain induced mRNA of these cytokines, and the induction appeared to be at the transcriptional level. When PBMC were stimulated with lipopolysaccharide (LPS), however, ouabain suppressed the production of IL-6 and TNF-α. Thus, cardiac glycosides may have different effects on the production of cytokines among individuals with versus those without immune activation. In other recent experiments in a murine model of EMCV-induced myocarditis, digoxin in high doses increased the mortality of the animals, as well as the extent of myocardial necrosis, amount of cellular infiltration, and production of intracardiac IL-1β and TNF-α [34]. The shorter survival did not seem attributable to direct toxicity, since none of the uninfected mice treated with digoxin, 10 mg/kg, died. In our previous study, 1 mg/kg of ouabain protected against LPS-induced lethal toxicity in mice, and suppressed circulating IL-6 and TNF-α [33]. However, 1 mg/kg of digoxin increased myocardial IL-1β and TNF-α in viral myocarditis. Thus, digitalis may have different effects on heart diseases caused by bacterial or viral infection as a result of its variable modulation of cytokines production. The results of this study suggests that digoxin exacerbates viral myocarditis, and that its use in high doses is contraindicated in patients suffering from CHF due to viral myocarditis.

We have also reported that amlodipine had a protective effect against myocardial injury in an animal model of heart failure due to viral myocarditis, and that its therapeutic effect may be partially attributable to inhibition of overproduction of nitric oxide [35]. Inducible nitric oxide is a type of calcium-independent nitric oxide synthase, and its inhibition is probably by inhibition of the cytokine production which mediates the induction of nitric oxide synthase. In a recent study from our laboratory, amlodipine inhibited the ouabain-induced production of IL-1α, IL-1β, and IL-6 in a concentration-dependent manner [36]. An earlier study had suggested that the mechanism of ouabain-induced production of cytokines was calcium dependent [33]. Thus, amlodipine may block calcium entry into mononuclear cells. The mechanism of its inhibition of cytokine production remains to be clarified.

Denopamine

Denopamine, is an orally active, selective β1-adrenergic agonist, which has no catecholamine moiety in its chemical structure. We found that denopamine directly suppressed LPS-induced TNF-α production from murine spleen cells. In splenic tissue, TNF-α is mainly synthesized by macrophages and lymphocytes. Agents that act via β_1-adrenoceptors inhibit LPS-induced TNF-α production from the promonocytic leukemia cell line THP-1 by increasing intracellular cyclic AMP levels. On the other hand, lymphocytes have β_2- but no β_1-adrenergic receptors. Since denopamine does not increase cyclic AMP via β_2-adrenergic receptors, even in a dose of 100 μmol/L, it probably does not act on lymphocytes through their β_2-receptors. To determine whether the effect of denopamine on TNF-α is mediated by β_1-adrenoceptors, the selective β_1-antagonist metoprolol was administered with denopamine. Metoprolol significantly blocked the effect of denopamine. Thus, denopamine seems to inhibit LPS-induced TNF-α production by macrophages via β_1-adrenoceptors in murine spleen cells [37]. We have also shown, in our murine model of viral myocarditis, that denopamine inhibits TNF-α production in the heart. When we examined the effects of denopamine combined with metoprolol in our *in vivo* model, metoprolol blocked the action of denopamine. Denopamine significantly prolonged survival and attenuated myocardial lesions [37]. These results suggest that the beneficial effects of denopamine are partially attributable to the suppression of TNF-α production.

Amiodarone

Amiodarone is now widely used to prevent life-threatening ventricular arrhythmias in patients with CHF. Although amiodarone did not reduce mortality in large-scale clinical trials, a significant reduction was measured in the combined endpoints of cardiac death and worsening heart failure [38]. When human PBMCs were cultured with amiodarone in the presence of LPS, cytokine levels in the culture supernatants were significantly reduced [39]. Since amiodarone blocks the inward rectifier K^+ channel, the inhibition of the K^+ current mediated T cell activation may be involved in this effect.

Interleukin-10

Current concepts of the immune responses focus on the cross-regulation between the two types of helper T cell. T helper type 1 (Th1) cells produce proinflammatory cytokines and contribute to cell-mediated immunity. The Th2-associated cytokines augment humoral immunity. The cytokines produced by one type of helper T cell regulate the others. The Th2-associated cytokine IL-10 has a variety of immunomodulatory properties involving the inhibition of Th1 cells, macrophage function, and the production of proinflammatory cytokines. IL-10 inhibits the inflammatory response by inhibiting the activation of NF-κB through preservation of IκBα. Recent reports have suggested that the profound immunosuppression associated with IL-10 may be effective against rejection of transplanted organ, immune complex diseases, and sepsis [40,41], and clinical trials of IL-10 have been carried out in patients with these conditions.

We have studied the effects of recombinant human IL-10 (rhIL-10) fully active on mouse cells, in a murine experimental model of heart failure caused by the EMCV. The survival in mice treated with rhIL-10 was significantly higher than in the control group. RhIL-10 treatment attenuated myocardial lesions, and suppressed TNF-α and IL-2 in the heart. RhIL-10 treatment had little effect on myocardial virus concentrations. The expression levels of myocardial iNOS mRNA was significantly decreased in the group treated with rhIL-10. These findings provide new insights into the *in vivo* effects of IL-10 on viral infection, and suggest a therapeutic effect of IL-10 in viral myocarditis. This study showed that IL-10 administration suppressed inflammation without altering virus replication, suggesting that it does not impair the host defense against intracellular pathogens *in vivo*. In this model of viral myocarditis, administration of IL-12 [42], and IFN-γ [43], also lowered mortality and attenuated myocardial injury. However, these results did not allow determining whether the beneficial effects on viral myocarditis were associated with a predominant response of Th1 or Th2. At this point, they merely point to the important role of these cytokines in the immune response and to their potential clinical applications. Exogenous cytokines or neutralizing antibodies influence several effectors of immune responses *in vivo*, including the induction or suppression of other endogenous cytokines. In addition, it has been reported that IL-10 acts in a Th-subset-independent fashion. A simple Th1–Th2 dichotomy may not explain the mechanisms of viral myocarditis. It has been recognized that the immune system may be inherently toxic to the host, and that the negative regulation of an immune response prevents the toxicity caused by excessive inflammation. This study shows that IL-10 may be a key regulatory cytokine protecting the organism against dangerous inflammatory responses.

Endothelin antagonists

An increase in circulating endothelin (ET)-1 has been reported in patients with CHF, and higher concentrations have been measured in the failing left ventricle than in plasma. In our animal model of heart failure, extensive inflam-mation develops in the heart, and myocardial and plasma ET-1 levels increased in parallel with the progression of myocardial injury [44]. The finding of higher ET-1 concentrations in myocardium than in plasma suggests that the heart is a major ET-1-producing organ in myocarditis. Our immunohistochemical studies were performed to identify the cellular origin of ET-1. While we found ET-1 to be localized in failing cardiac myocytes, as observed in previous studies, infil-trating mononuclear cells were also positive for ET-1, a finding specific of this model. However, tissue ET-1 had already risen by day 5 after virus inoculation, when few infiltrating cells were present. Therefore, myocytes and endothelial cells seem to produce ET-1 mostly before cellular infiltration occurs.

The recent development of specific endothelin receptor antagonists enables the study of important physiological and pathophysiological roles of endothelins, and of their receptors. Little information is available, however, regarding the effects of ET-1 receptor antagonists in acute myocarditis. Bosentan, a mixed ET$_A$ and ET$_B$ endothelin receptor antagonist, was chosen for our experiments because of recent conflicting results obtained with the continuous intravenous infusion of BQ-123, which reduced infarct size in dogs, versus that FR13937, which had no effects in rabbits. We hypothesized that mixed ET$_A$ and ET$_B$ endothelin receptor antagonism would be more effective in limiting myocardial injury since both ET$_A$ and ET$_B$ receptors are present in arterial and venous smooth muscle and in cardiac tissue, and since coronary vasoconstriction via ET$_B$ receptors had been demonstrated. Treatment with bosentan, was associated with a lower heart weight/body weight ratio, and lower histological scores for myocardial necrosis and cellular infil-tration, suggesting that ET-1 plays an important pathophysiologic role in viral myocarditis. Treatment with bosentan had a cardioprotective effect without modifying viral replication.

Acknowledgments

This work was supported, in part, by a research grant from the Japanese Ministry of Health and Welfare and a Grant-in-Aid for General Scientific Research from the Japanese Ministry of Education, Science and Culture. We would like to thank Drs Y. Sato, T. Shioi, Y. Kihara, Y. Furukawa, K. Ono, R. Nishio, A. Iwasaki for collaborative works and Ms. Y. Okazaki and Ms. S. Sakai for preparing the manuscript.

References

1. Sasayama S, Matsumori A, Kihara Y. New insights into the pathophysiological role for cytokines in heart failure. *Cardiovasc Res* 1999;42:557–564.

2. Levine B, Kalman J, Mayer L, Fillit HM, Packer M. Elevated circulating levels of tumor necrosis factor in severe chronic heart failure. *N Engl J Med* 1990;323:236–241.

3. Matsumori A, Yamada T, Suzuki H, Matoba Y, Sasayama S. Increased circulating cytokines in patients with myocarditis and cardiomyopathy. *Br Heart J* 1994;72:561–566.

4. Kubota T, McNamara DM, Wang JJ, Trost M, McTiernan CF, Mann DL, Feldman AM. Effects of tumor necrosis factor gene polymorphisms on patients with congestive heart failure. VEST Investigators for TNF Genotype Analysis. Vesnarinone Survival Trial. *Circulation* 1998;97:2499–2501.

5. MacGowan GA, Mann DL, Kormos RL, Feldman AM, Murali S. Circulating interleukin-6 in severe heart failure. *Am J Cardiol* 1997;79:1128–1131.

6. Sato Y, Takatsu Y, Kataoka K, Yamada T, Taniguchi R, Sasayama S, Matsumori A. Serial circulating concentrations of c-reactive protein, interleukin (IL)-4, and IL-6 in patients with acute left heart decompensation. *Clin Cardiol* 1999;22:811–813.

7. Matsumori A. Animal models: Pathological findings and therapeutic considerations. In: Banatvala JE, ed. *Viral infection of the heart.* Kent: Edward Arnold, London, 1993:110–137.

8. Matsumori A. Molecular and immune mechanisms in the pathogenesis of cardiomyopathy—Role of viruses, cytokines, and nitric oxide. *Jpn Circ J* 1997;61:275–291.

9. Kyu B, Matsumori A, Sato Y, Okada I, Chapman NM, Tracy S. Cardiac persistence of cardioviral RNA detected by the polymerase chain reaction in a murine model of dilated cardiomyopathy. *Circulation* 1992;86:522–530.

10. Matsumori A, Yamada T, Kawai C. Immunomodulating therapy in viral myocarditis: Effects of tumor necrosis factor, interleukin 2 and anti-interleukin-2 receptor antibody in an animal model. *Eur Heart J* 1991;12(Suppl D):203–205.

11. Yamada T, Matsumori A, Sasayama S. Therapeutic effects of anti-tumor necrosis factor-α antibody on the murine model of viral myocarditis induced by encephalomyocarditis virus. *Circulation* 1994;89:846–851.

12. Shioi T, Matsumori A, Sasayama S. Persistent expression of cytokine in the chronic stage of viral myocarditis in mice. *Circulation* 1996;94:2930–2937.

13. Jaattela M. Biology of disease: Biologic activities and mechanisms of action of tumor necrosis factor-alpha/cachectin. *Lab Invest* 1991;64:724–742.

14. Inoko M, Kihara Y, Morii I, Fujiwara H, Sasayama S. Transition from compensatory hypertrophy to dilated, failing left ventricles in Dahl salt-sensitive rats. *Am J Physiol* 1994;267:H2471–H2482.

15. Shioi T, Matsumori A, Kihara Y, Inoko M, Ono K, Iwanaga Y, Yamada T, Iwasaki A, Matsushima K, Sasayama S. Increased expression of interleukin-1β and monocyte chemotactic and activating factor (MCAF)/monocyte chemoattractant protein-1 (MCP-1) in the hypertrophied and failing heart with pressure overload. *Circ Res* 1997;81:664–671.

16. Aukrust P, Ueland T, Muller F, Andreassen AK, Nordoy I, Aas H, Kjekshus J, Simonsen S, Froland SS, Gullestad L. Elevated circulating levels of C-C

chemokines in patients with congestive heart failure. *Circulation* 1998;97:1136–1143.

17. Damås JK, Gullestad L, Ueland T, Solum NO, Simonsen S, Froland SS, Aukrust P. CXC-chemokines, a new group of cytokines in congestive heart failure—possible role of platelets and monocytes. *Cardiovasc Res* 2000;45:428–436.

18. Matsumori A, Furukawa Y, Hashimoto T, Yoshida A, Ono K, Shioi T, Okada M, Iwasaki A, Nishio R, Matsushima K, Sasayama S. Plasma levels of the monocyte chemotactic and activating factor/monocyte chemoattractant protein-1 are elevated in patients with acute myocardial infarction. *J Mol Cell Cardiol* 1997;29:419–423.

19. Sasayama S, Okada M, Matsumori A. Chemokines and cardiovascular diseases. *Cardiovasc Res* 2000;45:267–269.

20. Okada M, Matsumori A, Ono K, Furukawa Y, Shioi T, Iwasaki A, Matsushima K, Sasayama S. Cyclic stretch upregulates production of interleukin-8 and monocyte chemotactic and activating factor/monocyte chemoattractant protein-1 in human endothelial cells. *Arterioscler Thromb Vasc Biol* 1998;18:894–901.

21. Bozkurt B, Kribbs SB, Clubb FJ Jr., Michael LH, Didenko VV, Hornsby PJ, Seta Y, Oral H, Spinale FG, Mann DL. Pathophysiologically relevant concentrations of tumor necrosis factor-α promote progressive left ventricular dysfunction and remodeling in rats. *Circulation* 1998;97:1382–1391.

22. Ono K, Matsumori A, Shioi T, Furukawa Y, Sasayama S. Cytokine gene expression after myocardial infarction in rat hearts. Possible implication in left ventricular remodeling. *Circulation* 1998;98:149–156.

23. Ono K, Matsumori A, Furukawa Y, Igata H, Shioi T, Matsushima K, Sasayama S. Prevention of myocardial reperfusion injury in rats by an antibody against monocyte chemotactic and activating factor/monocyte chemoattractant protein-1. *Lab Invest* 1999;79:195–203.

24. Furukawa Y, Matsumori A, Ohashi N, Shioi T, Ono K, Harada A, Matsushima K, Sasayama S. Anti-monocyte chemoattractant protein-1/monocyte chemotactic and activating factor antibody inhibits neointimal hyperplasia in injured rat carotid arteries. *Circ Res* 1999;84:306–314.

25. Finkel MS, Oddis CV, Jacob TD, Watkins SC, Hattler BG, Simmons RL. Negative inotropic effects of cytokines on the heart mediated by nitric oxide. *Science* 1992;257:387–389.

26. Ungureanu-Longrois D, Balligand JL, Kelly RA, Smith TW. Myocardial contractile dysfunction in the systemic inflammatory response syndrome: role of a cytokine-inducible nitric oxide synthase in cardiac myocytes. *J Mol Cell Cardiol* 1995;27:155–167.

27. Matsumori A, Ono K, Sato Y, Shioi T, Nose Y, Sasayama S. Differential modulation of cytokine production by drugs: Implications for therapy in heart failure. *J Mol Cell Cardiol* 1996;28:2491–2499.

28. Matsumori A, Okada I, Shioi T, Furukawa Y, Nakamura T, Ono K, Iwasaki A, Sasayama S. Inotropic agents differentially inhibit the induction of nitric oxide synthase by endotoxin in cultured macrophages. *Life Sci* 1996;59:L121–L125.

29. Iwasaki A, Matsumori A, Yamada T, Shioi T, Wang W, Ono K, Nishio R, Okada M, Sasayama S. Pimobendan inhibits the production of proinflammatory cytokines and gene expression of inducible nitric oxide synthase in a murine model of viral myocarditis. *J Am Coll Cardiol* 1999;33:1400–1407.

30. Asea A, Kraeft SK, Kurt-Jones EA, Stevenson MA, Chen LB, Finberg RW, Koo GC, Calderwood SK. HSP70 stimulates cytokine production through a CD14-dependant pathway, demonstrating its dual role as a chaperone and cytokine. *Nat Med* 2000;6:435–442.

31. Baldwin AS Jr. The NF-κB and I-κB proteins: New discoveries and insights. *Annu Rev Immunol* 1996;14:649–681.

32. Baeuerle PA, Baichwal AV. NF-κB as a frequent target for immunosuppressive and anti-inflammatory molecules. *Adv Immunol* 1997;65:111–137.

33. Matsumori A, Ono K, Nishio R, Igata H, Shioi T, Matsui S, Furukawa Y, Iwasaki A, Nose Y, Sasayama S. Modulation of cytokine production and protection against lethal endotoxemia by the cardiac glycoside ouabain *Circulation* 1997;96:1501–1506.

34. Matsumori A, Igata H, Ono K, Iwasaki A, Miyamoto T, Nishio R, Sasayama S. High doses of digitalis increase the myocardial production of proinflammatory cytokines and worsen myocardial injury in viral myocarditis: A possible mechanism of digitalis toxicity. *Jpn Circ J* 1999;63:934–940.

35. Wang WZ, Matsumori A, Yamada T, Shioi T, Okada I, Matsui S, Sato Y, Suzuki H, Shiota K, Sasayama S. Beneficial effects of amlodipine in a murine model of congestive heart failure induced by viral myocarditis: A possible mechanism through inhibition of nitric oxide production. *Circulation* 1997;95:245–251.

36. Matsumori A, Ono K, Nishio R, Nose Y, Sasayama S. Amlodipine inhibits the production of cytokines induced by ouabain. *Cytokine* 2000;12:294–297.

37. Nishio R, Matsumori A, Shioi T, Wang W, Yamada T, Ono K, Sasayama S. Denopamine, a β1-adrenergic agonist, prolongs survival in a murine model of congestive heart failure induced by viral myocarditis. Suppression tumor necrosis factor-α production in the heart. *J Am Coll Cardiol* 1998;32:808–815.

38. Massie BM, Fisher SG, Radford M, Deedwania PC, Singh BN, Fletcher RD, Singh SN. Effect of amiodarone on clinical status and left ventricular function in patients with congestive heart failure. CHF-STAT Investigators. *Circulation* 1996;93:2128–2134.

39. Matsumori A, Ono K, Nishio R, Nose Y, Sasayama S. Amiodarone inhibits production of tumor necrosis factor-α by human mononuclear cells. A possible mechanism for its effect in heart failure. *Circulation* 1997;96:1386–1389.

40. Shanley TP, Schmal H, Friedl HP, Jones ML, Ward PA. Regulatory effects of intrinsic IL-10 in IgG immune complex-induced lung injury. *J Immunol* 1995;154:3454–3460.

41. Furukawa Y, Becker G, Stinn JL, Shimizu K, Libby P, Mitchell RN. Interleukin-10 (IL-10) augments allograft arterial disease: paradoxical effects of IL-10 in vivo. *Am J Pathol* 1999;155:1929–1939.

42. Shioi T, Matsumori A, Nishio R, Ono K, Kakio T, Sasayama S. Protective role of interleukin-12 in viral myocarditis. *J Mol Cell Cardiol* 1997;29:2327–2334.

43. Yamamoto N, Shibamori M, Ogura M, Seko Y, Kikuchi M. Effects of intranasal administration of recombinant murine interferon-γ on murine acute myocarditis caused by encephalomyocarditis virus. *Circulation* 1998;97:1017–1023.

44. Ono K, Matsumori A, Shioi T, Furukawa Y, Sasayama S. Contribution of endothelin-1 to myocardial injury in a murine model of myocarditis. Acute effects of bosentan, an endothelin receptor antagonist. *Circulation* 1999;100:1823–1829.

9. The Effect of Cytokines on Cardiac Allograft Function: Tumor Necrosis Factor-α: A Mediator of Chronic Injury

Alex Perez-Verdia, Sonny J. Stetson, Susan McRee, Wojciech Mazur, Michael M. Koerner, and Guillermo Torre-Amione

From the Gene and Judy Campbell Laboratories for Cardiac Transplant Research, The Winters Center for Heart Failure Research, and The DeBakey Heart Center at The Methodist Hospital and Baylor College of Medicine Houston, Texas

Introduction

Cardiac transplantation has evolved as the treatment of choice for the patient with advanced heart failure. However, the long-term survival of heart transplant recipients is limited by the development of complications associated with the immune response against the graft or complications that result from long-term use of immunosuppressive therapy. Despite the fact that cardiac transplantation represents the only treatment modality that radically alters the prognosis of the terminally ill heart failure patient, the function of the transplanted heart is not normal. For example, only 27% of heart transplant recipients are able to return to work full-time; while their functional class and exercise tolerance is better than prior to transplantation, it is not normal [1]. The mechanisms for abnormal graft function are the rapid progression of coronary arteriopathy and the development of left ventricular hypertrophy, which eventually leads to cardiac failure. In this review, we will discuss the potential effects of acute and chronic injury by cytokines expressed in the allograft.

The immune response against the heart: Acute Cardiac Injury

The clinical manifestations of acute rejection and the effects on contractile function are typified by the following clinical case. A 37 year old man 6 months post-heart transplantation has acute cellular rejection as defined by a high cellular score grade IIIB or IV of the ISHLT criteria. He presented with acute pulmonary edema and severe depression of left ventricular systolic function. However, after treatment with aggressive immunosuppressive therapy, left ventricular function normalized. Two weeks after treatment he underwent repeat endomyocardial biopsy that demonstrated no evidence of cellular rejection.

This clinical presentation that is typical of the acute rejection process suggests that the mechanism of decreased contractile function is not cell destruction. Allogeneic tissues elicit a vigorous reaction characterized by the release of cytokines and injury that may result from direct cell-target contact. During acute allograft rejection, both of these processes occur and the myocardium may be acutely exposed to an increasing number of cytokines as well as to the direct cell injury that results from the interaction of cytotoxic T cells in contact with myocardial cells [2–5]. Acute allograft rejection is associated with reversible myocardial dysfunction, and the reversible nature of this process suggests that the acute contractile dysfunction is not likely the result of direct cytotoxic T cell-target contact that results in myocyte cell death, (Fig. 1). Alternatively, the most likely explanation for the phenomenon of acute contractile dysfunction in the setting of acute rejection is the effect on the contractile state of the heart by the large number of cytokines that are released in the setting of acute rejection. The evidence to support these concepts can be summarized as follows: 1) Acute rejection is associated with the appearance of various cytokines in the graft and in the periphery [6–8], 2) Acute rejection is characterized by reversible negative inotropic effects; the resolution of acute allograft dysfunction in the setting of acute rejection is usually associated with normalization of ejection fraction, 3) Cytotoxic T cells destroy cells by the release of pore-forming proteins and cause irreversible cell damage [2,9], 4) The acute release of cytokines induces negative inotropic effects that are reversible [10–12]. It is important to emphasize that during acute rejection there is a massive and rapid increase in infiltrating cells that produce a large and diverse number of cytokines. However, even at lower levels of rejection, cardiac allografts contain persistently abnormal levels of cytokines and, in particular, of TNFα [13]. In the next section, we will discuss

Douglas L. Mann. *THE ROLE OF INFLAMMATORY MEDIATORS IN THE FAILING HEART.*
Copyright © 2001. Kluwer Academic Publishers. Boston. All rights reserved.

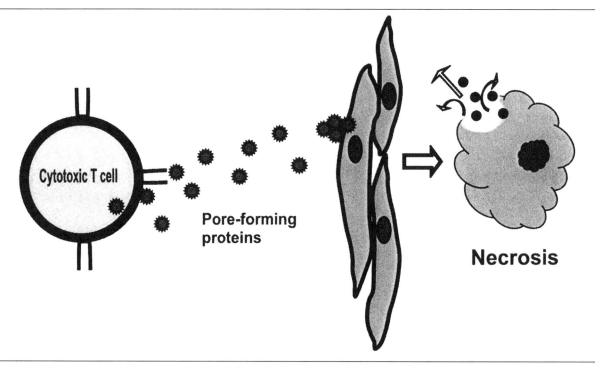

Fig. 1.   *Immune injury against cardiac allografts. Cytotoxic T cells release cytokines in response to alloantigen (cardiac cell) as well as secrete pore-forming proteins that are capable of causing cell membrane damage and irreversible cell destruction. The effect of the combination of these two pathways of injury results in reversible contractile dysfunction as well as some degree of irreversible injury leading to scar and fibrosis.*

the potential effects of persistent low-level expression of TNFα on cardiac function.

Acute versus chronic cytokine injury

The acute effects of cytokines may be different from those associated with long-term expression of cytokine in the myocardium. Experimentally, it is clear that acute exposure of myocytes to either IL-6 or TNFα causes reversible inotropic effects; however, there is no evidence to suggest that the negative inotropic effects are maintained chronically or that chronic low levels of TNFα lead to negative inotropic effects in vivo or in vitro. Indeed, cytokine receptors are usually down regulated following receptor binding [14,15] and this may partially explain the differences in contractile function in acute versus chronic cytokine exposures. To address these issues further we will concentrate our discussion on the effects of TNFα on cardiac function.

The mechanisms by which TNFα mediates negative inotropic effects are not clearly defined but involve the reduction of intracellular calcium [10] and the induction of nitric oxide that in turn decreases the contractile state of the cell [11,16]. However, all experimental conditions in which cytokines and in particular TNFα have been demonstrated to reduce contractility are in the setting of acute short-term experimental condi-

tions and therefore there is no evidence that chronic exposure of the myocardium to TNFα directly causes altered contractility.

Another important observation on the role of TNFα in cardiac allografts is that it appears to be chronically expressed. In a previous report from our group, we found that in random endomyocardial biopsies of patients from 1 week to 8 years following transplantation, we were able to detect TNFα in solubilized endomyocardial biopsy specimens of heart transplant recipients that showed no evidence of rejection [13]. These findings did not represent serial observations on individual patients; however, they strongly suggested that TNFα was persistently expressed in the myocardium in the setting of normal ventricular function. Therefore, it follows that during chronic TNFα exposure contractile function can be maintained.

We have taken these hypotheses further and have measured cardiac TNFα levels in normal controls, heart transplant recipients with normal systolic function, and in patients with end-stage heart failure and depress systolic function. As shown in Figure 2, we found that intra-cardiac TNFα levels were high in all three groups and therefore, there was no direct correlation between cardiac TNFα levels and contractile function. These data indicate that in chronic settings of myocardial TNFα expression, contractile function can be main-

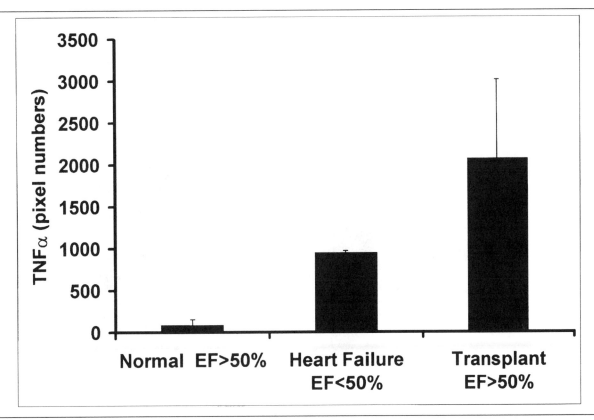

Fig. 2. *High levels of intra-cardiac TNFα can be found on patients with preserved left ventricular function. Intra-cardiac TNFα levels were determined by semi-quantitative immunohistochemistry on patients with end-stage heart failure and depressed LV function, normal controls and heart transplant recipients with normal LV systolic function. TNFα levels were high on heart failure and heart transplant recipients and were undetectable in the normal controls.*

tained. But clearly, the presence of TNFα in the heart is abnormal since normal myocardium from various experimental animals as well as in humans does not contain TNFα [15,17].

Potential effects of chronic TNFα expression in cardiac allografts

Cardiac function in the transplanted heart is affected by rejection, allograft associated atherosclerosis and by the rapid development of hypertrophy and fibrosis [18,19]. While there are increasing numbers of reports that describe the mechanisms of immune mediated cardiac injury and graft atherosclerosis [20–22], very little is known about the mediators responsible for hypertrophy and fibrosis that contribute to the development of diastolic dysfunction in cardiac allografts. The importance of recognizing the mechanisms of diastolic dysfunction in transplant myocardium is emphasized by the clinical observations that demonstrate that heart transplant recipients that manifest Doppler based echocardiographic features of diastolic abnormalities are at a higher risk of premature death [23]. The difficulty in studying hypertrophy in the trans-

plant setting is that a large number of patients develop hypertension and are under treatment with immunosuppressive therapy that may be important in the development of hypertrophy. In a small set of observations in an attempt to control for these variables, we determined the degree of left ventricular hypertrophy in heart transplant recipients and lung transplant recipients at 12 months following transplantation. The study population had similar degrees of hypertension and patients were treated with cyclosporine-based immunosupression. We found that 12 months following transplantation, left ventricular mass was significantly higher in the heart transplant population in comparison to the lung transplant group. This observation suggests that the immune response against the graft in heart transplant recipients may partially contribute to hypertrophy; clearly, neither hypertension nor drugs were sufficient to explain the differences in hypertrophy among the heart and lung transplant recipients, (Fig. 3).

Based on these clinical observations coupled with the fact that TNFα, a cytokine capable of inducing hypertrophy is persistently expressed in transplant myocardium, we have suggested that

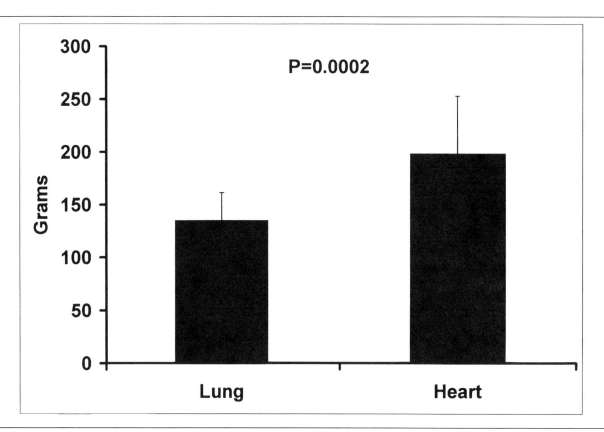

Fig. 3. *Left ventricular mass at 12 months on lung and heart transplant recipients. Left ventricular mass was determined by 2-D echocardiography 12 months following transplantation on heart (n = 9) and lung transplant recipients (n = 18). Both groups of patients were treated with triple based immuno-suppression and had similar degrees of hypertension. LV mass was significantly higher in the heart recipient population.*

persistent TNFα expression causes hypertrophy following cardiac transplantation.

In further support of this hypothesis are the striking similarities between the phenotype of transgenic mice that over-express TNFα in cardiac restricted manner and human transplant myocardium: 1) The myocardium in both conditions contains inflammatory infiltrates and develops hypertrophy [24,25], 2) At early stages of development, cardiac TNFα transgenic mice maintain normal systolic function in the presence of TNFα just like cardiac allografts, (Dr. D. E. Mann, personal communication) and finally, 3) TNFα transgenic mice and cardiac transplant recipients die prematurely.

To further define the role of TNFα in the development of post-transplant hypertrophy, we are conducting a clinical trial in heart transplant recipients in whom we plan to define the effect of TNFα antagonism on the development of post-transplant hypertrophy. The EFECT (effect of etanercept on cardiac transplants) trial will randomize patients within 2 weeks of transplantation to either placebo or tri-weekly subcutaneous injections of etanercept (a chimeric soluble TNFα receptor that blocks the biological effects of

TNFα) for 6 months. We will compare the gain in left ventricular mass among the two study groups. The results of this study will provide the experimental basis to conduct a large-scale study to define the full clinical benefit of chronic TNFα suppression in cardiac allografts.

References

1. Brann WM, Bennett LE, Keck BM, Hosenpud JD. Morbidity, functional status, and immunosuppressive therapy after heart transplantation: an analysis of the joint International Society for Heart and Lung Transplantation/United Network for Organ Sharing Thoracic Registry. *J Heart Lung Transplant* 1998; 17(4):374–382.
2. Wagoner LE, Zhao L, Bishop DK, Chan S, Xu S, Barry WH. Lysis of adult ventricular myocytes by cells infiltrating rejecting murine cardiac allografts. *Circulation* 1996;93(1):111–119.
3. Lange LG, Schreiner GF. Immune mechanisms of cardiac disease. *N Engl J Med* 1994;330(16):1129–1135.
4. Hastillo A, Willis HE, Hess ML. The heart as a target organ of immune injury. *Curr Probl Cardiol* 1991;16(6):377–442.
5. Barry WH. Mechanisms of immune-medicated myocyte injury. *Circulation* 1994;89(5):2421–2432.

6. Suzuki J, Isobe M, Yamazaki S, Horie S, Okubo Y, Sekiguchi M. Sensitive diagnosis of cardiac allograft rejection by detection of cytokine transcription in situ. *Cardiovasc Res* 1998;40(2):307–313.

7. Saber LT, Aliberti JC, Silva JS, Rossi MA, Ferraz AS. Chemokine profile during allogeneic heart transplant rejection. *Transplant Proc* 1999;31(7):2978–2981.

8. Chollet-Martin S, Depoix JP, Hvass U, Pansard Y, Vissuzaine C, Gougerot-Pocidalo MA. Raised plasma levels of tumor necrosis factor in heart allograft rejection. *Transplant Proc* 1990;22(1):283–286.

9. Frisman DM, Fallon JT, Hurwitz AA, Dec WG, Kurnick JT. Cytotoxic activity of graft-infiltrating lymphocytes correlates with cellular rejection in cardiac transplant patients. *Hum Immunol* 1991;32(4):241–245.

10. Yokoyama T, Vaca L, Rossen RD, Durante W, Hazarika P, Mann DL. Cellular basis for the negative inotropic effects of tumor necrosis factor-alpha in the adult mammalian heart. *J Clin Invest* 1993;92(5):2303–2312.

11. Finkel MS, Oddis CV, Jacob TD, Watkins SC, Hattler BG, Simmons RL. Negative inotropic effects of cytokines on the heart medicated by nitric oxide. *Science* 1992;257(5068):387–389.

12. Bozkurt B, Kribbs SB, Clubb FJ, Jr., Michael LH, Didenko VV, Hornsby PJ, Seta Y, Oral H, Spinale FG, Mann DL. Pathophysiologically relevant concentrations of tumor necrosis factor-alpha promote progressive left ventricular dysfuction and remodeling in rats. *Circulation* 1998;97(14):1382–1391.

13. Torre-Amione G, MacLellan W, Kapadia S, Weilbaecher D, Farmer J, Young J, Mann D. Tumor necrosis factor-alpha is persistently expressed in cardiac allografts in the absence of histological or clinical evidence of rejection. *Transplant Proc* 1998;30(3):875–877.

14. Holtmann H, Wallach D. Down regulation of the receptors for tumor necrosis factor by interleukin 1 and 4 beta-phorbol-12-myristate-13-acetate. *J Immunol* 1987;139(4):1161–1167.

15. Torre-Amione G, Kapadia S, Lee J, Durand JB, Bies RD, Young JB, Mann DL. Tumor necrosis factor-alpha and tumor necrosis factor receptors in the failing human heart. *Circulation* 1996;93(4):704–711.

16. Horton JW, Maass D, White J, Sanders B. Nitric oxide modulation of TNF-alpha-induced cardiac contractile dysfunction is concentration dependent. *Am J Physiol Heart Circ Physiol* 2000;278(6):H1955–H1965.

17. Kapadia S, Lee J, Torre-Amione G, Birdsall HH, Ma TS, Mann DL. Tumor necrosis factor-alpha gene and protein expression in adult feline myocardium after endotoxin administration. *J Clin Invest* 1995;96(2):1042–1052.

18. Rowan RA, Billingham ME. Pathologic Changes in the long-term transplanted heart: a morphometric study of myocardial hypertrophy, vascularity, and fibrosis. *Hum Pathol* 1990;21(7):767–772.

19. Imakita M, Tazelaar HD, Rowan RA, Masek MA, Billingham ME. Myocyte hypertrophy in the transplanted heart. A morphometric analysis. *Transplantation* 1987;43(6):839–842.

20. Young JB. Cardiac allograft arteriopathy: an ischemic burden of a different sort. *Am J cardiol* 1992;70(16):9F–13F.

21. Gao SZ, Alderman EL, Schroeder JS, Silverman JF, Hunt SA. Accelerated coronary vascular disease in the heart transplant patient: coronary arteriographic findings. *J Am Coll Cardiol* 1988;12(2):334–340.

22. Costanzo-Nordin MR. Cardiac allograft vasculopathy: relationship with acute cellular rejection and histocompatibility. *J Heart Lung Transplant* 1992;11(3 Pt 2):S90–103.

23. Alvarez R, McNamara D, Rosemblum W, Muralli S, Bozkurt B. Restricted physiology late after transplantation adversely affects survival. *Circulation* 1997;SI-6:376.

24. Bryant D, Decker L, Richardson J, Shelton J, Franco F, Peshock R, Thompson M, Giroir B. Cardiac failure in transgenic mice with myocardial expression of tumor necrosis factor-alpha [see comments]. *Circulation* 1998;97(14):1375–1381.

25. Kubota T, McTiernan CF, Frye CS, Slawson SE, Lemster BH, Koretsky AP, Demetris AJ, Feldman AM. Dilated cardiomyopathy in transgenic mice with cardiac-specific overexpression of tumor necrosis factor-alpha. *Circ Res* 1997;81(4):627–635.

10. The Role of Anti-Cytokine Therapy in the Failing Heart

Anita Deswal, MD, Arunima Misra, MD, and
Biykem Bozkurt, MD

Winters Center for Heart Failure Research, Cardiology Section,
Department of Medicine, Veterans Administration Medical Center
and Baylor College of Medicine, Houston, Texas 77030

Clinical and experimental studies have identified the important role of 'neurohormones' in the progression of heart failure. This has led to the utilization of agents that antagonize the activation of neurohormonal systems (the renin angiotensin system and the adrenergic system) as effective therapy in patients with heart failure. Recently, another class of biologically active molecules, the proinflammatory cytokines, has also been implicated as a mediator in the progression of heart failure. Some of the current interest in understanding the role of proinflammatory cytokines in heart failure relates to the following observations. First, many aspects of the syndrome of heart failure can be explained by the *known* biological effects of these molecules. When expressed at sufficiently high concentrations, cytokines mimic certain aspects of the heart failure phenotype, including left ventricular (LV) dysfunction, pulmonary edema, LV remodeling, fetal gene expression and cardiomyopathy [1,2]. Second, elevated circulating levels of cytokines, in particular, tumor necrosis factor (TNF), have consistently been identified in patients with advanced heart failure [3]. Third, several studies suggest that there is increasing cytokine elaboration in direct relation to the severity of the disease process [4–7]. Fourth, increasing levels of TNF may be associated with increased mortality in patients with congestive heart failure [5]. Thus, analogous to elevated levels of neurohormones, TNF levels may be predictive of the functional class and clinical outcome in patients with heart failure and may represent a biochemical mechanism that is responsible for producing symptoms in patients with heart failure. Just as benefits have been seen with agents that antagonize the neurohormonal system, it is reasonable to ask whether antagonizing cytokines may lead to clinical improvements in patients with heart failure. The majority of studies addressing this issue have focused on the modulation of TNF synthesis and TNF bioactivity, and our discussion, therefore, will summarize the results of studies designed to regulate the production and

biological action of this cytokine. However, before doing so, it is instructive to obtain an understanding of cytokine bioactivity and cytokine receptors and to review the regulation of TNF biosynthesis in the heart.

Cytokine bioactivity

As shown in Figure 1, in order to interpret the biological activity of any cytokine, it is extremely important to know the concentration of the cytokine that one is measuring, the concentration of the receptors on which the cytokine is acting, as well as the presence and/or absence of any circulating antagonists or agonists for the particular cytokine of interest. Thus, it is possible to detect circulating levels of cytokines in disease states (e.g. heart failure) that lack biological activity because the cytokine is bound to and inactivated by its cognate circulating soluble receptors.

Cytokine receptors

The effects of cytokines are thought to be initiated by their binding to specific receptors that exist on the membranes of most mammalian cell types, including the adult cardiac myocyte. TNF binds to one of two TNF receptors, a lower affinity ($K_d = 2-10 \times 10^{-10}$) 55 kD 'type 1 receptor' (also called TNFR1) and a higher affinity ($K_d = 2-10 \times 10^{-11}$) 75 kD 'type 2 receptor' (also called TNFR2). Intracellular signaling through TNF receptors occurs as a result of TNF induced cross-linking, or oligomerization, of the receptors. Both TNFR1 and TNFR2 share homology in their extracellular domains, which each contain a characteristic repeated cysteine consensus motif. However, no significant homology exists between the intracellular domains of TNFR1 and TNFR2, suggesting that each receptor has distinct modes of signaling and cellular function. Studies have identified the presence of both types of TNF receptors in non-failing [8] and failing human myocardium [9]. Both TNF receptor subtypes have been immunolocalized to the adult human cardiac myocyte. Although, the exact functional significance of TNFR1 and TNFR2 in the heart is not presently clear, it appears that most of the

---

*Dr. Deswal has received a Clinical Research Career Development Award (CRCD #712B) from the Veterans Affairs Cooperative Studies Program.

Douglas L. Mann. THE ROLE OF INFLAMMATORY MEDIATORS IN THE FAILING HEART.
Copyright © 2001. Kluwer Academic Publishers. Boston. All rights reserved.

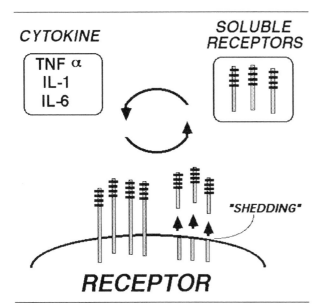

Fig. 1. *Cytokine Bioactivity. When interpreting the biological activity of any cytokine it is important to know the concentration of the cytokine that one is measuring, the concentration of the receptors on which the cytokine is acting, as well as the presence and/or absence of any circulating antagonists or agonists for the particular cytokine of interest. (Modified from Bozkurt et al [45])*

deleterious effects of TNF are coupled to activation of TNFR1, whereas activation of TNFR2 appears to exert protective effects in the heart. However, it should be emphasized that the entire range of effects that are downstream from TNFR1 and TNFR2 mediated signaling in cardiac myocytes, still remains to be determined. TNFR1 activation mediates negative inotropic effects [8] (through activation of the neutral sphingomyelinase pathway [10]), cardiac myocyte apoptosis, and increased HSP 72 expression [11]. In contrast, type 2 TNF receptor (TNFR2) activation appears to protect the myocyte against hypoxic stress and ischemic injury. An interesting observation about the biology of TNF receptors is that mammalian cells appear to 'shed' TNF receptors following exposure to a variety of different stimuli, including TNF, lipopolysaccharide, okadaic acid or phorbol esters [12–14]. Once the type 1 (TNFR1) and type 2 (TNFR2) TNF receptors are proteolytically cleaved from the cell membrane, they exist in the circulation as circulating 'soluble' receptors (referred to as a sTNFR1 and sTNFR2, respectively). Both soluble receptors retain their ability to bind ligand, and to inhibit the cytotoxic effects of TNF in cell culture. While the definitive biological role for these soluble TNF binding proteins *in vivo* is not known, it has been postulated that they may serve as 'biological buffers' which are capable of rapidly

neutralizing the highly cytotoxic activities of TNF. Recent experiments have shown that sTNFRs are sufficient to both block as well as reverse the negative inotropic effects of TNF [15]. It has also been hypothesized that soluble TNF receptors may stabilize TNF as a homotrimer, and hence increase TNF bioactivity *relative* to unstabilized TNF which will dissociate into inactive monomers [16]. Indeed, elevated levels of sTNFR2 have been shown to correlate with an adverse clinical outcome in patients hospitalized for heart failure [4]. Taken together, these data raise the interesting possibility that sTNFRs may provide an immediate short term benefit to the host by buffering the potentially untoward effects of TNF; however, in the long-term elevated levels of these receptors may be maladaptive by stabilizing biologically active TNF and slowly releasing it into the circulation.

TNF biosynthesis in the heart

Presently available evidence suggests that in the normal adult heart, TNF gene and protein expression are self-limited and occur only in relation to a superimposed environmental stress. This is supported by the following experimental observations. First, neither TNF mRNA nor TNF protein appear to be constitutively expressed in the unstressed adult mammalian heart [17–19]. Second, both TNF mRNA and protein are rapidly synthesized by the heart in response to an appropriate stressful stimulus [17–19]. Third, once TNF mRNA biosynthesis is initiated, myocardial TNF mRNA levels rapidly return toward baseline following removal of the inciting stress [18]. Thus, strategies aimed at either blocking TNF gene expression, or hastening degradation of TNF mRNA may be effective in modulating TNF expression in the failing heart.

Strategies for anti-cytokine therapy

Experimental studies have shown that agents that raise cAMP levels, such as pentoxifylline, amrinone and milrinone, prevent TNF mRNA accumulation, largely by blocking the transcriptional activation of TNF [20–23]. Dexamethasone, which is thought to primarily suppress TNF biosynthesis at the translational level, may also block TNF biosynthesis at the transcriptional level [24]. When initially translated, TNF exists as a 26 kDa propeptide with 76 extra amino acids appended to the amino terminus. This propeptide is efficiently cleaved by a matrix metalloproteinase which exists in cell membranes [25], to form the mature 17 kDa TNF peptide. Recently, specific inhibitors of matrix metalloproteinases have been shown to prevent the proteolytic cleavage of the 26 kDa form of TNF from the membrane [25–27], thus preventing the 17 kDa form of TNF from being released into the peripheral circulation. Thalidomide (α-N-pthalimidoglutarimide) is another class of drug that may be useful in suppressing TNF production. Thalidomide selectively inhibits TNF production in monocytes [28]. It appears to reduce TNF levels by enhancing mRNA degradation [29]. Since the teratogenic and sedative properties of thalidomide may limit its clinical utility, thalidomide analogues which have more potent TNF lowering properties, and at the same time appear to be non teratogenic, are being developed.

On the basis of the above observations, a number of studies attempting to suppress cytokine production in patients with heart failure, have employed strategies that are designed to block TNF expression at the transcriptional or translational levels. One of the earliest studies that raises the possibility that suppression of proinflammatory cytokines may play an important role in heart failure was performed by Parrillo and colleagues [30]. They randomly assigned 102 patients to either treatment with prednisone (60 mg per day) or placebo. Following three months of therapy, they observed an increase in ejection fraction of $\geq 5\%$ in 53% of the patients receiving prednisone, whereas only 27% of the controls had a significant improvement in ejection fraction (p = 0.005). Overall, the mean ejection fraction increased $4.3 \pm 1.5\%$ in the prednisone group, as compared with $2.1 \pm 0.8\%$ in the control group (p = 0.054). The patients were then categorized prospectively into two separately randomized subgroups. 'Reactive' patients had fibroblastic or lymphocytic infiltration or immunoglobulin deposition on endomyocardial biopsy, a positive gallium scan, or an elevated erythrocyte sedimentation rate and 'nonreactive' patients, had none of these features. At three months, 67% of the reactive patients who received prednisone had improvement in LV function, as compared with 28% of the reactive controls (p = 0.004). In contrast, nonreactive patients did not improve significantly with prednisone (p = 0.51). Although specific cytokine levels were not measured in this study, their data suggest that patients with idiopathic dilated cardiomyopathy may have some improvement when given a high dose of prednisone daily.

Another potentially important pharmacological method for suppressing TNF production is through the use of agents that elevate cAMP levels, such as dobutamine. Short-term dobutamine infusion has been shown to suppress TNF production [31]. One can then speculate that one of the mechanisms for the sustained benefit of

intravenous infusions of dobutamine [32,33] may be through suppression of proinflammatory cytokines such as TNF. However, this speculation is not supported by a recent publication, in which it was shown that treatment with either intravenous dobutamine or milrinone (which also raises cAMP and might therefore be expected to decrease TNF levels) had no effect in terms of decreasing circulating TNF levels despite clinical improvement [34]. In contrast to the findings with respect to TNF, Deng and colleagues reported that interleukin-6 (IL-6) levels increased in patients with NYHA class III–IV heart failure after treatment with dobutamine [35]. However, the mechanism for this increase in IL-6 levels was not elucidated.

More encouraging results with respect to modulating TNF levels through alterations in intracellular cAMP levels have been reported recently by Wagner et al. [36,37] and Sliwa et al. [38] Wagner and colleagues showed that adenosine was sufficient to block lipolysaccharide induced TNF production in cultured neonatal and adult rat myocytes, as well as in slices of human myocardium obtained from explanted failing human hearts. The effect of adenosine could be mimicked by PD-125944, a selective A_2 receptor agonist (which is known to increase cAMP levels), or forskolin, and antagonized by DPMX, an A_2-selective antagonist. However, adenosine was only able to block TNF production if given before lipopolysaccharide challenge. Adenosine has also been shown to suppress intramyocardial TNF levels in an *ex vivo* model of ischemia reperfusion in the rat, as well as improve post-ischemic myocardial function [39]. More recently Sliwa and associates studied the effects of pentoxifylline in patients with dilated cardiomyopathy and NYHA class II–III heart failure. All patients were receiving concurrent therapy with digitalis, diuretics and ACE inhibitors for four months. A total of 14 patients received pentoxifylline at a dose of 400 mg three times daily and an equal number received placebo. The primary endpoint of the six month study were NYHA functional class and left ventricular function. Four patients died as a result of progressive pump dysfunction during the six month study period, all in the placebo group. At the end of six months there was an improvement in functional class in the pentoxifylline group, whereas there was functional deterioration in the placebo group. At six months there was a significant increase in the ejection fraction (from 22.3 ± 9.0 [S.D.] to 38.7 ± 15.0 [S.D.]) in the pentoxifylline group, whereas there was no significant change in the placebo group. There was, however, no change in the LV end-diastolic dimension in either group. An important observa-

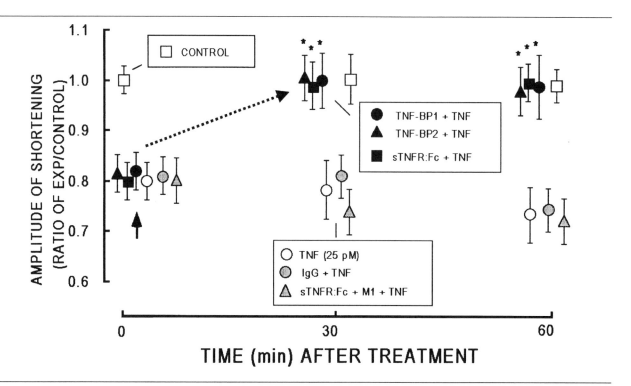

Fig. 2. *'Cell Rescue' using soluble TNF receptor. Treatment of isolated cardiac myocytes with diluent alone had no effect on the contractile properties of the isolated cardiac myocytes (open squares), whereas treament of cardiac myocytes with 25 pM TNF (open circle) resulted in a 20% depression in cell shortening, which was stable over the 60-minute course of the study. Starting at time 0 (solid arrow), cardiac myocytes that had been treated previously with TNF were exposed to neutralizing concentrations of sTNFR1 (solid circle), sTNFR2 (solid triangle), or STNFR:Fc (solid square). As shown, the addition of a neutralizing concentration of sTNFR1, sTNFR2 or sTNFR:Fc resulted in a reversal (dashed arrow) of the negative inotropic effects of TNF within 30 muinutes (p < 0.05 compared to the respective values for these cells at time 0). (Reproduced with permission from Kapadia et al [15], the American Journal of Physiology).*

tion was that TNF levels fell significantly (p < 0.002) from 6.5 ± pg/ml to 2.1 ± 1.0 pg/ml in the pentoxifylline group, whereas there was no significant change in the TNF levels in the placebo group. Thus, it appears that modulation of TNF levels via agents that alter intracellular cAMP levels, thus blocking transcriptional activation of TNF, may be a useful strategy for altering cytokine levels in heart failure. However, it is unclear whether the levels of intracellular cAMP levels that are necessary to suppress cytokine production will also be proarrhythmic in patients with heart failure.

Mohler and colleagues employed a different strategy to alter cytokine levels in patients with heart failure [40]. These authors examined the effects of amlodipine on circulating levels of TNF and IL-6 in a subset analysis of patients enrolled in the PRAISE trial [41]. They observed that although treatment with amlodipine had no effect on TNF levels, there was a statistically significant decrease in IL-6 levels following 24 weeks of treatment [40].

Targeted anti-cytokine therapy in heart failure

Instead of suppressing cytokine production in the setting of disease states, an alternative strategy is to prevent TNF and/or other cytokines from binding to their cognate receptors. In the case of TNF, early studies showed that antibodies directed at either TNFR1 and/or TNFR2 led to activation, as opposed to abrogation, of TNFR mediated signaling, presumably as a result of cross-linking of the TNF receptors by the anti-TNFR antibodies. For this reason, strategies designed to block TNF receptors have not proven to be effective in terms of modulating the deleterious effects of TNF. A second, more successful, approach has utilized circulating soluble TNF receptors as 'decoys' to prevent TNF from binding to its cognate receptors on cell surface membranes. That cytokines might be antagonized by their soluble cognate receptors relates back to the concept of 'cytokine bioactivity'. As shown in Figure 1, when soluble TNF receptors bind TNF, they are capable of preventing TNF from

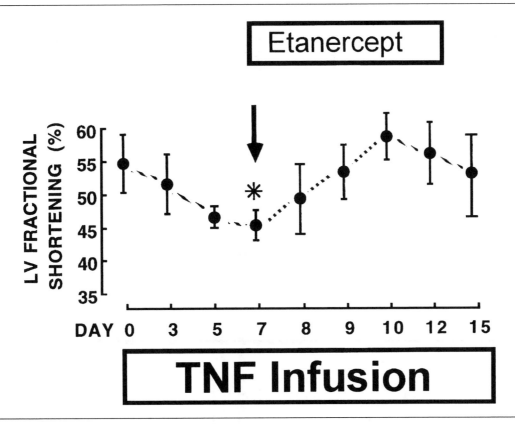

Fig. 3. *Myocardial rescue using a TNF antagonist. To determine whether the effects of TNF on LV function could be antagonized with a soluble TNF receptor, rats that had received a continuous infusion of 2.5 μg/kg/min TNF for 7 days were treated with a single s.c. dose of TNFR:Fc. The figure depicts the changes in 2-D echocardiographically determined LV fractional shortening following the administration of TNFR:Fc (arrow). The solid horizontal bars indicate the days that circulating levels of TNFR:Fc were detectable in the peripheral circulation (* = p < 0.05 compared to control values at day 0) (Reproduced with permission from Bozkurt et al. [1] the American Heart Association).*

binding to TNF receptors on cell surface membranes. Previous studies in isolated contracting cardiac myocytes have shown that both the type 1 and the type 2 TNF receptor were sufficient to reverse the negative inotropic effects of TNF (Fig. 2) [15]. In this *in vitro* study neutralizing concentrations of monomeric p55 (sTNFR1) and p75 TNF (sTNFR2) receptors, as well as a dimeric p75 chimeric fusion protein, were sufficient to block, as well as reverse (i.e. 'rescue') the negative inotropic effects of TNF within 30 min. The dimeric p75 chimeric fusion protein consists of two of the extracellular p75 TNF receptors fused in duplicate to the Fc portion of the IgG$_1$ molecule (TNFR:Fc, etanercept). Also, once the negative inotropic effects of TNF were reversed by the addition of TNF soluble receptors, there was no subsequent deterioration of myocyte contractile function over a 3.5 hour period of observation [15]. These *in vitro* findings were then tested in an *in vivo* study in rats [1]. TNF was infused at

pathophysiologically relevant concentrations (≈80–100 U/ml) in order to provoke a heart failure phenotype (i.e. left ventricular dilation and left ventricular dysfunction). Figure 3 shows that infusion of TNF *in vivo* resulted in a ≈20% decrease in left ventricular function. However, when the animals were treated with a single subcutaneous injection of the chimeric fusion protein TNFR:Fc, there was a time-dependent improvement in left ventricular function within 24 h, and a complete restoration of left ventricular function to normal levels within 48 h after the administration of TNFR:Fc. Thus targeted anti-cytokine therapy was sufficient to reverse the deleterious effects of TNF *in vivo* [1].

Recently, Deswal and colleagues have utilized targeted anti-cytokine therapy as a novel approach to treating patients with moderate to advanced heart failure [42]. These investigators studied 18 patients with NYHA class III heart failure, who were receiving standard therapy for heart failure, including digitalis, diuretics and

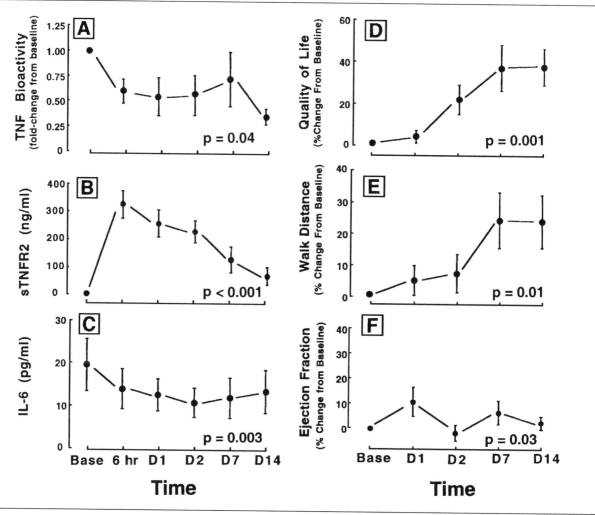

Fig. 4.   *Biological and functional effects of etanercept in patients with moderate to advanced heart failure. Panels A–C (left) show the effects of etanercept on TNF bioactivity and on levels of sTNFR2 and IL-6. Panels D–F (right) show the changes in clinical endpoints for the pateints who received either the 4 mg/m^2 or 10 mg/m^2 of etanercept. (Reproduced with permission from Deswal et al. [42] the American Heart Association).*

angiotensin converting enzyme inhibitors. Patients were randomized into a double-blind dose escalation study designed to examine the safety and efficacy of targeted anti-cytokine therapy with etanercept. Patients received placebo (6 patients) or an escalating dose (1, 4 or 10 mg/m^2) of etanercept (12 patients), given as a single intravenous infusion. Safety parameters and patient functional status were assessed at baseline and at days 1, 2, 7 and 14. The investigators reported that there were no significant side effects nor clinically significant changes in laboratory indices. Moreover, they reported that there was a significant decrease in TNF bioactivity (Fig. 4A) and a significant overall increase in quality of life scores, 6 minute-walk distance and ejection fraction in the cohort that received 4 or 10 mg/m^2 of etanercept (Figs. 4D–4F), whereas

there was no significant change in these parameters in the placebo group. Thus, in this study a single intravenous infusion of etanercept appeared to have salutary effects in patients with heart failure. The results of this phase I study must be regarded as provisional because of the relatively small numbers of patients and the relatively short duration of follow-up.

More recently, in order to evaluate the safety of repeated doses of etanercept, a larger phase I study was conducted at three different sites. Forty-seven patients with NYHA Class III–IV heart failure were treated with biweekly subcutaneous injections of etanercept 5 mg/m^2 (n = 16), etanercept 12 mg/m^2 (n = 15) or placebo (n = 16) in a double-blind, randomized study for 3 months [43]. The investigators reported that both doses of etanercept were well tolerated over the 3 month period. For the patients who received 5 and $12 \, \text{mg/m}^2$ etanercept, there were improvements in left ventricular ejection fraction and left ventricular volumes measured by echocardiography [44]. There was a trend towards improvement in the clinical composite score. The improvements were more pronounced in the group that received $12 \, \text{mg/m}^2$ of etanercept [43].

Whether the beneficial effects that were observed with etanercept in these two studies [42,43] can be sustained when etanercept is given repeatedly over longer periods of time and in larger patient populations is now being addressed in two ongoing multicenter clinical trials. The *R*andomized *E*tanercept *N*orth *Amer*I*can Strategy to Study Antago*N*ism of Cyto-kin*E*s (RENAISSANCE) is currently enrolling patients with NYHA class II–IV heart failure in the U.S. and the *R*esearch into *E*tanercept Cyto-kine Antagonism in *V*entricula*r* Dysfunction (RECOVER), a companion study, is enrolling patients in Europe and Australia.

Conclusion

In the present review we have focused on the rationale to develop anti-cytokine strategies for the treatment of heart failure. In addition, we have reviewed the experimental and clinical literature which suggests that circulating cytokines can be antagonized effectively through a variety of different 'targeted' strategies. While it is too early to predict whether modulating cytokine levels will translate into clinical improvements in morbidity and mortality for patients with heart failure, there is now a growing body of evidence which suggests that anti-cytokine therapy may represent a new approach for the treatment of patients with heart failure.

References

1. Bozkurt B, Kribbs S, Clubb FJ Jr, Michael LH, Didenko VV, Hornsby PJ, Seta Y, Oral H, Spinale FG, Mann DL. Pathophysiologically relevant concentrations of tumor necrosis factor-α promote progressive left ventricular dysfunction and remodeling in rats. *Circulation* 1998;97:1382–1391.
2. Kubota T, McTiernan CF, Frye CS, Slawson SE, Koretsky AP, Demetris AJ, Feldman AM. Dilated cardiomyopathy in transgenic mice with cardiac specific overexpression of tumor necrosis factor-alpha. *Circ Res* 1997;81:627–635.
3. Mann DL. Cytokines as mediators of disease progression in the failing heart. In: Hosenpud JD, Greenberg BH, ed. *Congestive Heart Failure*. Philadelphia: Lippincott Williams & Wilkins, 2000:213–232.

4. Ferrari R, Bachetti T, Confortini R, Opasich C, Febo O, Corti A, Cassani G, Visioli O. Tumor necrosis factor soluble receptors in patients with various degrees of congestive failure. *Circulation* 1995;92:1479–1486.
5. Torre-Amione G, Kapadia S, Benedict CR, Oral H, Young JB, Mann DL. Proinflammatory cytokine levels in patients with depressed left ventricular ejection fraction: a report from the studies of left ventricular dysfunction (SOLVD). *J Am Coll Cardiol* 1996;27:1201–1206.
6. Testa M, Yeh M, Lee P, Fanelli R, Loperfido F, Berman JW, LeJemtel TH. Circulating levels of cytokines and their endogenous modulators in patients with mild to severe congestive heart failure due to coronary artery disease or hypertension. *J Am Coll Cardiol* 1996;28:964–971.
7. MacGowan GA, Mann DL, Kormas RL, Feldman AM, Murali S. Circulating interleukin-6 in severe heart failure. *Am J Cardiol* 1997;79:1128–1131.
8. Torre-Amione G, Kapadia S, Lee J, Bies RD, Lebovitz R, Mann DL. Expression and functional significance of tumor necrosis factor receptors in human myocardium. *Circulation* 1995;92:1487–1493.
9. Torre-Amione G, Kapadia S, Lee J, Durand JB, Bies RD, Young JB, Mann DL. Tumor necrosis factor-α and tumor necrosis factor receptors in the failing human heart. *Circulation* 1996;93:704–711.
10. Oral H, Dorn GW, II, Mann DL. Sphingosine mediates the immediate negative inotropic effects of tumor necrosis factor-α in the adult mammalian cardiac myocyte. *J Biol Chem* 1997;272:4836–4842.
11. Krown KA, Page MT, Nguyen C, Zechner D, Gutierrez V, Comstock KL, Glembotsi CC, Quintana PJE, Sabbadini RA. Tumor necrosis factor alpha-induced apoptosis in cardiac myocytes: involvement of the sphingolipid signaling cascade in cardiac cell death. *J Clin Invest* 1996;98:2854–2865.
12. Olsson I, Lantz M, Nilsson E, Peetre C, Thysell H, Grubb A, Adolf G. Isolation and characterization of a tumor necrosis factor binding protein from urine. *Eur J Haematol* 1989;42:270–275.
13. Engelmann GL, Novick D, Wallach D. Two tumor necrosis factor-binding proteins purified from human urine. *J Biol Chem* 1990;265:1531–1536.
14. Brakebusch C, Nophar Y, Kemper O, Engelmann H, Wallach D. Cytoplasmic truncation of the p55 tumour necrosis factor (TNF) receptor abolishes signalling, but not induced shedding of the receptor. *EMBO J* 1992;11:943–950.
15. Kapadia S, Torre-Amione G, Yokoyama T, Mann DL. Soluble tumor necrosis factor binding proteins modulate the negative inotropic effects of TNF-α *in vitro*. *Am J Physiol* 1995;37:H517–H525.
16. Aderka D, Engelmann H, Maor Y, Brakebusch C, Wallach D. Stabilization of the bioactivity of tumor necrosis factor by its soluble receptors. *J Exp Med* 1992;175:323–329.
17. Giroir BP, Johnson JH, Brown T, Allen GL, Beutler B. The tissue distribution of tumor necrosis factor biosynthesis during endotoxemia. *J Clin Invest* 1992;90:693–698.
18. Kapadia S, Lee JR, Torre-Amione G, Birdsall HH, Ma TS, Mann DL. Tumor necrosis factor gene and

protein expression in adult feline myocardium after endotoxin administration. *J Clin Invest* 1995;96: 1042–1052.

19. Kapadia S, Oral H, Lee J, Nakano M, Taffet GE, Mann DL. Hemodynamic regulation of tumor necrosis factor-α gene and protein expression in adult feline myocardium. *Circ Res* 1997;81:187–195.

20. Zabel P, Schade FU, Schlaak M. Inhibition of Endogenous TNF Formation by Pentoxifylline. *Immunbiol* 1993;187:447–463.

21. Zabel P, Greinert U, Entzian P, Schlaak M. Effects of pentoxifylline on circulating cytokines (TNF and IL-6) in severe pulmonary tuberculosis. In: Fiers W, Buurman WA, ed. *Tumor Necrosis Factor: Molecular and Cellular Biology and Clinical Relevance*. Basel: S. Karger, 1993:178–181.

22. Dezube BJ, Pardee AB, Chapman B, Beckett LA, Korvick JA, Novick WJ, Chiurco J, Kasdan P, Ahlers CM, Ecto LT, Crumpacker CS. Pentoxifylline decreases tumor necrosis factor expression and serum triglycerides in people with AIDS. *J Acq Immun Defic Syndrome* 1993;6:787–794.

23. Giroir BP, Beutler B. Effect of amrinone on tumor necrosis factor production in endotoxin shock. *Circ Shock* 1992;36:200–207.

24. Remick DG, Strieter RM, Lynch IJP, Nguyen D, Eskandari M, Kunkel SL. In vivo dynamics of murine tumor necrosis factor-α gene expression. Kinetics of dexamethasone-induced suppression. *Lab Invest* 1989;60:766–771.

25. Mohler KM, Sleath PR, Fitzner JN, Cerretti DP, Alderson M, Kerwar SS, Torrance DS, Otten-Evans C, Greenstreet T, Weerawarna K, Kronheim SR, Petersen M, Gerhart M, Kozlosky CJ, March CJ, Black RA. Protection against a lethal dose of endotoxin by an inhibitor of tumor necrosis factor processing. *Nature* 1994;370:218–220.

26. Gearing AJH, Beckett P, Christodoulou M, Churchill M, Clements J, Davidson AH, Drummond AH, Galloway WA, Gilbert R, Gordon JL, Leber TM, Mangan M, Miller K, Nayee P, Owen K, Patel S, Thomas W, Wells G, Wood LM, Woolley K. Processing of tumor necrosis factor-α precursor by metalloproteinases. *Nature* 1994;380:555–557.

27. McGeehan GM, Becherer JD, Bast RC, Boyer CM, Champion B, Connolly KM, Conway JG, Furdon P, Karp S, Kidao S, McElroy AB, Nicholas J, Pryzwansky M, Schoenen F, Sekut L, Truesdale A, Vergheses M, Warner J, Ways JP. Regulation of tumor necrosis factor-α by a metalloproteinase inhibitor. *Nature* 1994;370:558–561.

28. Sampaio EP, Sarno EN, Galilly R, Cohen ZA, Kaplan G. Thalidomide selectively inhibits tumor necrosis factor α production by stimulated human monocytes. *J Exp Med* 1991;173:699–703.

29. Moreira AL, Sampaio EP, Zmuidzinas A, Frindt P, Smith KA, Kaplan G. Thalidomide exerts its inhibitory action on tumor necrosis factor-alpha by enhancing messenger RNA degradation. *J Exp Med* 1993;177:1675–1680.

30. Parrillo JE, Cunnion RE, Epstein SE, Parker ME, Suffredini AF, Brenner M, Schaer GL, Palmeri ST, Cannon RO, Alling D, Wittes JT, Ferrans VJ, Rodriguez ER, Fauci AS. A prospective randomized controlled tiral of prednisone for dilated cardiomyopathy. *N Engl J Med* 1989;321:1061–1068.

31. Sindhwani R, Yuen J, Hirsch H, Tegguy A, Galvao M, Levato P, LeJemtel TH. Reversal of low flow state attenuates immune activation in severe decompensated congestive heart failure. *Circulation* 1993;88:I-255.

32. Leier CV, Huss P, Lewis RP, Unverferth DV. Drug-induced conditioning in congestive heart failure. *Circulation* 1982;65:1382–1387.

33. Unverferth DV, Magorien RD, Lewis RP, Leier CV. Long-term benefit of dobutamine in patients with congestive cardiomyopathy. *Am Heart J* 1980; 100:622–630.

34. Milani RV, Mehra MR, Endres S, Eigler A, Cooper S, Lavie CJ Jr, Ventura HO. The clinical relevance of circulating tumor necrosis factor-α in acute decompensated chronic heart failure without cachexia. *Chest* 1996;110:992–997.

35. Deng MC, Erren M, Lutgen A, Zimmermann P, Brisse B, Schmitz W, Assman G, Breithardt G, Scheld HH. Interleukin-6 correlates with hemodynamic impairment during dobutamine administration in chronic heart failure. *Int J Cardiol*. 1996;57: 129–134.

36. Wagner DR, Combes A, McTiernan CF, Sanders VJ, Lemster B, Feldman AM. Adenosine inhibits lipopolysacchide-induced cardiac expression of tumor necrosis factor-α. *Circ Res* 1998;82:47–56.

37. Wagner DR, McTiernan CF, Sanders VJ, Feldman AM. Adenosine inhibits lipopolysaccharide-induced secretion of tumor necrosis factor-α in the failing human heart. *Circulation* 1998;97:521–524.

38. Sliwa K, Skudicky D, Candy G, Wisenbaugh T, Sareli P. Randomized investigation of effects of pentoxifylline on left ventricular performance in idiopathic dilated cardiomyopathy. *Lancet* 1998;351:1091–1093.

39. Meldrum DR, Cain BS, Cleveland JC Jr, Meng X, Ayala A, Banerjee A, Harken AH. Adenosine decreases post-ischemic cardiac TNFα production: anti-inflammatory implications for preconditioning and transplantation. *Immunology* 1997;92:472–477.

40. Mohler ER III, Sorensen LC, Ghali JK, Schocken DD, Willis PW, Bowers JA, Cropp AB, Pressler ML. Role of cytokines in the mechanism of action of amlodipine: The PRAISE heart failure trial. *J Am Coll Cardiol* 1997;30:35–41.

41. Packer M, O'Connor CM, Ghali JK, Pressler ML, Carson PE, Belkin RN, Miller AB, Neuberg GW, Frid D, Wertheimer JH, Cropp AB, DeMets DL. Effect of amlodipine on morbidity and mortality in severe chronic heart failure. *N Engl J Med* 1996;335:1107–1114.

42. Deswal A, Bozkurt B, Seta Y, Parilti-Eiswirth S, Hayes FA, Blosch C, Mann DL. A phase I trial of tumor necrosis factor receptor (p75) fusion protein (TNFR:Fc) in patients with advanced heart failure. *Circulation* 1999;99:3224–3226.

43. Bozkurt B, Torre-Amione G, Soran OZ, Feldman AM, Blosch C, Warren M, Mann DL. Results of a phase I trial with tumor necrosis factor receptor (p75) fusion protein (Etanercept) in patients with heart

failure. *J Am Coll Cardiol* 1999;33:2 Suppl I, 1110–10.

44. Bozkurt B, Torre-Amione G, Deswal A, Soran OZ, Whitmore J, Warren M, Mann DL. Regression of left ventricular remodeling in chronic heart failure after treatment with enbrel (Etanercept, p75 TNF receptor Fc fusion protein). *Circulation* 1999;100:I, 105.

45. Bozkurt B, Shan K, Seta Y, Oral H, Mann DL. Tumor necrosis factor-α and tumor necrosis factor receptors in human heart failure. *Heart Fail Rev* 1996;1:211–219.

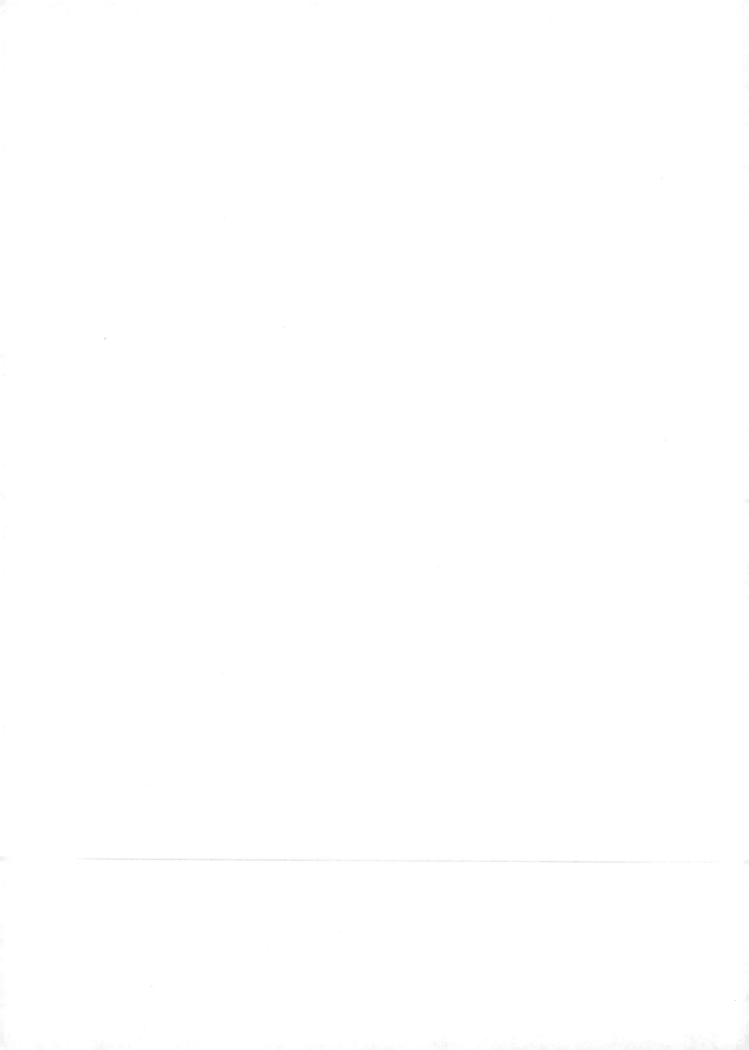

11. The Syndrome of Cardiac Cachexia

Stefan D. Anker, MD, PhD[1,2] and
Rakesh Sharma, BSc, MRCP[1]

[1]Clinical Cardiology, National Heart & Lung Institute, Imperial College School of Medicine, London, UK and [2]Franz Volhard Klinik (Charité, Campus Berlin-Buch) at Max Delbrück Centrum for Molecular Medicine, Berlin, Germany

Introduction

It has long been recognised that significant weight loss and wasting are important features of advanced chronic heart failure (CHF). This dates back 2300 years to the school of medicine of Hippocrates (about 460–370 BC) on the island of Cos: "The flesh is consumed and becomes water, ..., the shoulders, clavicles, chest and thighs melt away. This illness is fatal, ..." [1]. The term cachexia is of Greek origin, derived from the words *kakos* (i.e. bad) and *hexis* (i.e. condition). Cachexia is a process of muscle wasting and weight loss that occurs in several different chronic disorders and is also part of the aging process, being almost always associated with a poor prognosis.

Cardiac cachexia is a serious complication of CHF which, until relatively recently, has been little investigated [2]. Whether the process of weight loss in this condition is accompanied by a loss of cardiac muscle tissue has never been studied, and whether the distinction between peripheral and cardiac cachexia is necessary remains unanswered. The available knowledge concerning the presence of general weight loss in CHF patients, its pathogenesis (with particular emphasis on the immunological and neurohormonal abnormalities present in this condition), and the potential treatment strategies for cardiac cachexia will be reviewed.

Definition of cardiac cachexia

The problems of research into cardiac cachexia start with its definition. Although research groups have extensively investigated the wasting process in different conditions, there is still no consensus with regard to the best definition of cachexia. Body composition analyses with body fat and lean tissue estimation and anthropometric measurements (skinfold thickness, arm muscle circumference), calculations of predicted percent ideal mass matched for sex, age and height (e.g. using data of the Metropolitan Life Insurance Tables from 1959 [3]), scores including serum albumin concentrations, cell-mediated immunity changes, weight/height index or body mass index (BMI = weight/height^2) and the history of weight loss have all been used [4]. In heart failure studies, patients were classified 'malnourished' when the body fat content was $< 22\%$ in women and $< 15\%$ for men or when the percentage of ideal weight was $< 90\%$ [5]. Other groups defined CHF patients prospectively as 'cachectic' when the body fat content was $< 29\%$ (females) or $< 27\%$ (males) [6], or when the ideal body weight was $< 85\%$ [7] or even $< 80\%$ [8]. Additionally it is possible to characterise lean body mass by several different methods. These include studying urinary creatinine excretion rates, skeletal muscle protein turnover using labeled amino acids, body densitometry, bioelectrical impedance, or measurement of skeletal muscle size by means of magnetic resonance and computerised tomography [2]. Freeman and Roubenoff suggested in 1994 [9] that a documented loss of at least 10% of lean tissue should be used as the criteria to define cardiac cachexia. The disadvantages of such a definition are that many physicians may not have easy access to facilities that allow prospective measurement of lean body mass, that this definition is muscle focused without considering first that fat tissue replacement may be intact with no general weight loss and second that some patients may suffer principally from fat tissue loss with little or no lean tissue loss, and finally that this would cause fairly large additional costs.

It is important to note that the development of the cachectic state in CHF is a dynamic process that can only be proven by documented weight loss measured in a non-edematous state. Including weight loss as a criterion excludes patients who have a constitutionally low body weight. We suggest the use of a relatively wide definition of 'clinical cardiac cachexia': *In patients with CHF of at least 6 months duration without signs of other primary cachectic states (like cancer, thyroid disease, or severe liver disease), cardiac cachexia can be diagnosed when weight loss $> 7.5\%$ of the previous normal weight is observed.* Significant weight loss over a short time period may be cardiac

Douglas L. Mann. THE ROLE OF INFLAMMATORY MEDIATORS IN THE FAILING HEART.
Copyright © 2001. Kluwer Academic Publishers. Boston. All rights reserved.

cachexia, but obviously other causes of wasting (such as cancer and infection) need to be carefully considered and excluded [2].

The advantage of this definition is that it is simple and quickly applicable. In general the previous normal weight of a heart failure patient would be the average weight prior to the onset of heart disease (e.g. before a myocardial infarction, or before the diagnosis of idiopathic dilated cardiomyopathy) and on the time axis it would be important to note the last time point when the patient had this weight without being edematous. In some cases, particularly when patients suffer from mild to moderate heart failure over longer time periods, a few patients may develop obesity after the onset of heart failure, and one would need to take this (higher) weight as the previous normal weight. However, in our experience such patients are uncommon and are unlikely to subsequently develop cardiac cachexia.

It appears useful to differentiate cachectic patients into those that are severely cachectic (with $> 15\%$ weight loss, or $> 7.5\%$ weight loss and ideal body weight $< 85\%$) and patients with early or moderate cachexia (definition: > 7.5 to 15% weight loss, or $> 7.5\%$ weight loss and ideal weight 85%). Furthermore, it should be noted that the cut-off value of 7.5% weight loss for the definition of cardiac cachexia remains arbitrary. In fact, detailed analysis of the results from the Studies of Left Ventricular Dysfunction (SOLVD) trial suggest that $> 6\%$ weight loss may be considered clinically the optimal cut-off value as this most strongly predicts impaired survival [10].

Epidemiology

It is widely recognised that the prevalence of chronic heart failure (CHF) is increasing [11]. This has been attributed to improved survival in patients with coronary artery disease, the use of drug therapy prolonging life in patients with established CHF, and a strong correlation between CHF and age in populations with increasing longevity. The natural and perioperative morbidity and mortality of patients with cardiac cachexia is higher than that of non-cachectic patients [12]. The New York Heart Association (NYHA) class does not correlate with disease morbidity or mortality in cardiac cachexia. Cardiac cachexia also occurs in childhood in relation to malnutrition and/or malabsorption diseases, i.e. kwashiorkor or marasmus [13]. Nevertheless, to date there has been no comprehensive large scale study on the frequency and degree of body wasting in CHF. In our clinic, between June 1993 and May 1995, we performed the first prospective study of the frequency and

prognostic importance of cachexia in CHF patients using the definition given above. Amongst 171 consecutively assessed CHF patients (age 60 ± 11 years, mean $\pm$ SD; 17 female; treadmill peak oxygen consumption [VO$_2$] 17.5 ± 6.8 ml/kg/min; functional NYHA class I: n = 21, II: 63, III: 68, IV: 19), we identified 28 as being cachectic, i.e. 16% of our CHF outpatient population has cardiac cachexia [4]. The observed weight loss in these patients amounted to 9 to 36%, i.e. 6 to 30 kg, within the prior 0.5 to 13 years (average weight loss per year 6.0 ± 3.7 kg). The cachectic patients were found to have an 18 month mortality of 50%, which is worse than the prognosis for some forms of cancer (Fig. 1).

Detailed analyses of large clinical trials in CHF suggest that cardiac cachexia may be more common than previously thought. For example, in the SOLVD trial the incidence of weight loss $> 7.5\%$ was found to be as high as 35% of the study population over three years with the cross-sectional prevalence being 12–13% [10].

Etiology

Historically, three distinct mechanisms were thought to be responsible for the development of cardiac cachexia: a) malabsorption and metabolic dysfunction, b) dietary deficiency and c) loss of nutrients via the urinary or digestive tracts. Pittman and Cohen in 1964 were the first to analyse extensively the pathogenesis of the syndrome of cardiac cachexia [14]. They proposed the development of cellular hypoxia as being the principal pathogenic factor leading to less efficient intermediary metabolism, thereby producing increased catabolism (protein loss) and reduced

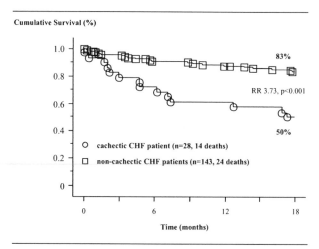

Fig. 1. *Kaplan–Meier plot for 18-month survival of 171 patients with chronic heart failure subgrouped according to cachexia. Adapted from [4].*

anabolism. Additionally, they suggested that anorexia and increased basal metabolic rate were closely related, potentially being the result of a lack of oxygen.

Little is known about the mechanisms of the transition from heart failure to cardiac cachexia. Anorexia can be related to heart failure via its main symptoms, i.e. fatigue and dyspnea, or via intestinal edema causing nausea and/or a protein losing gastroenteropathy. Additionally, anorexia may be iatrogenic as a side effect of drug therapy (e.g. digoxin, ACE inhibitors), and sodium restricted diets. To test this hypothesis Buchanan and colleagues performed a study in 1977 in 11 cachectic patients (NYHA class IV, mitral valve disease, pre- and postoperative assessment) [15]. They found marked anorexia—that was reversible—to be the most common cause of the cachectic state. Neither malabsorption (D-xylose absorption test) nor cellular hypoxia (assessed by lactate and pyruvate concentration) was of importance in their patients. In contrast it was recently demonstrated that elderly ambulatory patients with cardiac cachexia (mean age 76 years) showed evidence of fat malabsorption [16]. It has been argued that cardiac cachexia is due to gastrointestinal protein loss, but in 5-day stool collections the recovery radioactivity indicative of protein excretion (chromic chloride test) was similar in cachectic CHF patients as compared to healthy age- and sex-matched subjects (p = 0.9, [16]). It is not clear to what degree these results hold true for younger patients with cardiac cachexia.

In 1984, Braunwald suggested that patients with cardiac cachexia may have biventricular heart failure, and that a predominant right ventricular component could be more common in these patients [17]. Interestingly, increased right atrial pressure was the only independent predictor of malnutrition observed in 24 out of 48 investigated patients with severe CHF [5]. In this study cardiac index and pulmonary capillary wedge pressure had been similar in malnourished and well-nourished CHF patients. In contrast, MacGowan and colleagues [18] found in a comparison of 9 cachectic and 9 non-cachectic patients that were considered for heart transplantation (ideal weight $75 \pm 7\%$ vs $105 \pm 16\%$) no differences in right atrial pressure, pulmonary arterial pressure, pulmonary capillary wedge pressure, and pulmonary and peripheral vascular resistance, but cardiac output (p < 0.05) and cardiac index were worse in the cachectics (1.9 ± 0.4 vs $2.2 \pm 0.5 \, \text{l/min/m}^2$, p = 0.08). Simple starvation and anorexia are often considered to be the main cause of cardiac cachexia, but they would predominantly lead to a loss of fat tissue. Also they would cause reduced plasma albumin levels. Yet, cachectic CHF patients suffer from fat, muscle, and bone tissue loss (indicating the presence of a general wasting process), and albumin as well as liver enzyme levels were not decreased in the cachectic patients [19]. This would argue against a major contribution of starvation, anorexia, gastrointestinal malabsorption or liver synthetic dysfunction in these patients. The latter would also be expected to be present if right heart failure would indeed be dominant in cachectic CHF patients.

Physical inactivity and deconditioning have been suggested as being important for the muscle atrophy observed in many patients with CHF [20], but histological evidence suggests that the atrophy in states of reduced activity is significantly different from the muscle atrophy observed in CHF [21]. Therefore it seems unlikely that physical inactivity is of great importance in the genesis of cardiac cachexia. In 1994, Poehlman et al. demonstrated increased resting metabolic rates in stable patients with CHF as compared to controls [22]. When the same group recently studied cachectic CHF patients and compared them to non-cachectic patients and healthy control subjects [23], they found no evidence of increased resting metabolic rate in cachectic patients that may lead to the development of wasting per se. Rather they found a reduced resting metabolic rate in cachectics (-9.1% when compared to controls), and an increased resting metabolic rate in non-cachectics ($+10.9\%$ vs controls). Total daily energy expenditure and physical activity energy expenditure were also lower in the cachectic patients, but it is important to note that in this study relatively old subjects were investigated (mean age 73 years). Interestingly, the resting metabolic rate has been shown to correlate with increasing concentrations of catecholamines in older individuals [24]. Whether this holds true for heart failure patients is not known, although it seems likely.

Inflammatory cytokine activation

There is now considerable evidence to suggest that neurohormonal and immune mechanisms may play a central role in the pathogenesis of cardiac cachexia, which is likely to have a dramatic effect on the way that this condition is managed in the future [2]. The immune system is the body's natural defense mechanism against infection and other stresses. There are several different components to this system which interact with each other in a complex manner and may be involved in the development of cardiac cachexia [25]. In 1990 it was reported by Levine and colleagues that tumor necrosis factor alpha (TNF) is increased in patients in cardiac cachexia [7]. This was subsequently confirmed by other groups [6,26]. Using our definition of cardiac cachexia, we found that TNF plasma levels were primarily increased in cachectic CHF patients, being the strongest predictors of the degree of previous weight loss (Fig. 2) [19]. TNF is one of the key cytokines important to the development of catabolism together with interleukin-1 (IL-1), IL-6, Interferon-γ and transforming growth factor-β.

The main stimulus for the immune activation that is seen in CHF is not known and at present there are three main theories. One hypothesis is that the heart itself is the main source of inflammatory cytokines as it has been shown that the failing myocardium is capable of producing TNF [27]. The second hypothesis is that the bowel wall edema which occurs in CHF is responsible for bacterial translocation with subsequent endotoxin release and immune activation [28]. This hypothesis is strengthened by the fir~~ding that~~

there are elevated concentrations of endotoxin in patients during an acute edematous exacerbation, which can be normalised by diuretic therapy [29]. It has been proposed that acute venous congestion can lead to altered gut permeability for bacteria and endotoxin, which may subsequently enter the circulation and stimulate inflammatory cytokine activation. Alternatively, the third hypothesis that has been proposed is that hypoxia may be the stimulus for increased TNF production in CHF patients [30].

Inflammatory cytokines are known to have multiple effects, many of which can directly or indirectly contribute to body wasting in CHF. In animal experiments it has been shown that cachexia occurs when TNF producing tumor cells are implanted into skeletal muscle, whereas TNF producing cells implanted in the brain cause profound anorexia [31]. This shows firstly that

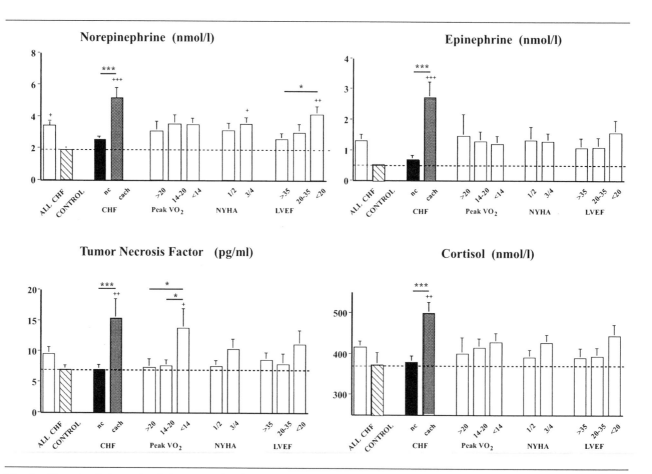

Fig. 2. *Norepinephrine, epinephrine, cortisol and tumor necrosis factor (TNF) plasma levels in 16 healthy controls and 53 patients with chronic heart failure (CHF). Patients are sub-grouped according to cachectic state (nc: non-cachectic, n = 37; cach: cachectic, n = 16); maximal oxygen consumption ([Peak VO$_2$], < 14 (n = 17) vs 14–20 (n = 24) vs > 20 ml/kg/min (n = 12)); functional New York Heart Association class ([NYHA], class 1/2 (n = 16) vs class 3/4 (n = 37)); and left ventricular ejection fraction ([LVEF], < 20 (n = 24) vs 20–35 (n = 17) vs > 35% (n = 12)). Data presented as mean ± SEM. P-values for Fisher's test are given if ANOVA showed significant inter-group variation. Symbols: *P < 0.05 for inter-group comparison, **P < 0.01 for inter-group comparison, ***P < 0.001 for inter-group comparison, +P < 0.05 vs controls, ++P < 0.01 vs controls, +++P < 0.001 vs controls, Adapted from [19].*

the site of production and action of TNF modifies its effect and secondly that increased levels of TNF may indeed play a causative role in the genesis of cachexia. TNF also can induce apoptosis, which may be important in the development of the cachectic state [25]. TNF also exerts effects on endothelial cells including rearrangement of the cytoskeleton, increased permeability to albumin and water, enhanced expression of activation antigens, induction of surface procoagulant activity and IL-1 release, and additionally TNF is known to reduce constitutive NO synthase mRNA in vascular endothelial cells [25]. These actions could all impair endothelial function. The strong inverse relationship between maximal peripheral blood flow and TNF levels in CHF patients could support the idea of detrimental effects of long term increased TNF effects [32].

TNF leads to an increase in the plasma concentrations of the hormone leptin in a dose dependent fashion [33]. Leptin, a product of the ob gene, acts centrally to decrease food intake and increase resting energy expenditure. Plasma levels of leptin have been shown to be elevated in patients with CHF [34], although it is doubtful that leptin is important for cardiac cachexia pathophysiology [35]. Interleukin-6, another pro-inflammatory cytokine which is elevated in CHF patients [36], has also been implicated in the etiology of wasting in CHF [2].

Recently, it has been demonstrated that elevated plasma levels of cytokines and soluble cytokine receptors significantly predict impaired survival in patients with CHF [37]. In particular, soluble TNF receptor 1 (sTNF-R1) levels appear to be the most accurate predictors of mortality, with the highest sensitivity and specificity amongst all immune parameters. The assessment of sTNF-R1 levels may therefore be of benefit in the stratification of CHF patients according to prognosis, thereby enabling high risk patients to be targeted more effectively.

CHF is associated not only with immune activation, but the elevation of other inflammatory markers which also relate adversely to prognosis [38]. There is a strong correlation between serum uric acid, an indicator of increased xanthine oxidase activity, and circulating markers of inflammation in patients with CHF (Fig. 3) [39]. Furthermore, serum uric acid appears to be an accurate and independent prognosticator in patients with CHF (unpublished data) which can be more easily and inexpensively assessed than cytokine levels.

Neuroendocrine abnormalities

A variety of secondary changes occur when heart failure becomes chronic (i.e. after 3 or 6 months) and are a response predominantly to the

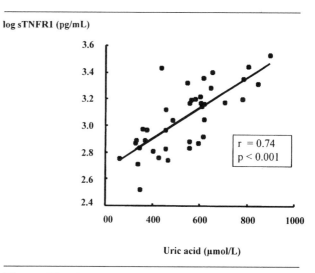

Fig. 3. *The relationship between serum uric acid and soluble TNF receptor-1 (sTNFR1) in 39 patients with CHF. Adapted from [39].*

impaired cardiac function, although some of these secondary changes may develop consequent upon the drugs used in the treatment of heart failure. These secondary changes include general neurohormonal activation with stimulation of the sympathetic nervous system, the renin-angiotensin-aldosterone-axis, and the natriuretic peptide system. Initially, these systems are thought to be beneficial, but eventually they contribute to increased vascular resistance and afterload, and ventricular enlargement and remodeling. According to the neurohormonal hypothesis [40], heart failure progresses due to activation of endogenous neurohormonal systems which exert deleterious effects on the heart and circulation. Several studies have found neurohormonal activation to be strongly related to mortality, but different hormones correlate only weakly with each other. Plasma norepinephrine is considered a marker of overall sympathetic activity and both norepinephrine and epinephrine can cause a catabolic metabolic shift [19].

Since the original observation in 1962 of increased catecholamines in CHF [41], no study had investigated catecholamine levels specifically in cachectic CHF patients until recently. When we stratified 53 CHF patients for presence of cachexia, peak VO$_2$, LVEF, and NYHA class, we found that cachectic CHF patients showed markedly increased norepinephrine and epinephrine levels, with non-cachectic CHF patients having near-normal levels (Fig. 2) [19]. None of the other subclassifications revealed significant differences between groups of CHF patients. Furthermore, aldosterone plasma levels and plasma renin activity were increased in patients with cardiac cachexia, although treatment with ACE inhibitors and diuretics and the time since diagnosis of CHF were similar [19]. This suggests a specific association between cachexia and sympathetic activation in CHF. Renin is a potent stimulator of the production of stress hormones such as angiotensin II and norepinephrine. Angiotensin II is capable of causing anorexia and wasting in animal models by reducing circulating insulin-like growth factor I (IGF-I) levels [42].

In patients with cardiac cachexia there is a significant relationship between indices of neuro-hormonal activation (such as levels of epinephrine and norepinephrine) and the impairment of cardiorespiratory reflex control [43]. Patients with cardiac cachexia have profound abnormalities in autonomic reflex control, as characterised by an abnormal profile of heart rate variability, and depressed baroreceptor sensitivity both of which are known to be associated with poor outcome and may contribute to the persistent neurohormonal activation in these patients. Catecholamines can contribute to the wasting state by a variety of different mechanisms. They can lead to a rise in basal metabolic rate in healthy subjects and an increase in resting energy expenditure in patients with CHF [44]. There appears to be a graded increase in resting metabolic rate according to NYHA class, which supports the hypothesis that the clinical severity of illness relates to the degree of the increase in resting energy demands [44].

Another hormone considered to be part of the general stress response with a catabolic action is cortisol. The cachectic patients in our study had a 2-fold increase of cortisol levels [19]. No other sub-grouping of the CHF patients revealed any significant effect on mean cortisol levels. In addition, the anabolic steroid dehydroepiandrosterone was lowest in cachectic CHF patients, suggestive of a catabolic/anabolic imbalance [19]. Interestingly, abnormalities of sex steroid metabolism in CHF are strongly and directly related to the immune activation seen in cachectic CHF patients [45].

Body composition alterations

Patients with CHF characteristically have evidence of muscle atrophy [46,47], being present in up to 68% of patients in certain studies [20]. Muscle weakness and early fatigue are two of the main symptoms experienced by CHF patients, and in the largest series reported to date (n = 101) we found muscle weakness and fatigue to occur mainly in patients with NYHA class 3 and 4 [48], and cachectic subjects [49]. A loss of lean body mass is known to predict prognosis in cancer and AIDS [50]. However, such a direct relationship has not as yet been documented in

CHF. A study in 27 patients with CHF and a mean weight 21% lower than normal subjects (weight loss itself was not documented) failed to show loss of fat tissue, but documented an average total body potassium decrease of 35% (measure of lean tissue independent of body water content) [51]. In these studies, neither clinical data, drug intake or humoral factors have been found to predict loss of muscle and fat tissue nor reduced bone mineral density in any group of heart failure patients.

When using documented weight loss as criterion to dichotomise CHF patients, it is found that cachectic CHF patients not only suffer from significant loss of lean tissue, but also have a gross reduction in fat tissue mass (i.e. energy reserves) and evidence of decreased bone mineral density (i.e. osteoporosis) [49]. Using dual energy x-ray absorptiometry, we [52] and others [23] could confirm, that cachectic CHF patients have a reduction in total body fat, lean tissue mass, and bone mineral density [53] as compared to non-cachectics and healthy controls. Considering the loss of muscle tissue (muscle quantity), it is certainly not surprising that cachectic CHF patients show greater muscle weakness than non-cachectic patients (both legs: 39% lower strength), but they also have a 16% reduction of strength per unit muscle, i.e. impaired muscle quality [49]. Additionally, the loss of muscle tissue is important as it, together with the impaired peripheral blood flow seen in CHF patients [54], contributes to the decreased oxidative capacity which is the main cause of the impaired exercise capacity of patients with heart failure.

The etiology of the body composition changes in cardiac cachexia is not entirely clear. Inflammatory cytokine and catabolic hormone levels in cachectic CHF patients are known to correlate significantly with the reduction of muscle, fat and bone tissue content in this disorder [55]. Alterations of the growth hormone/IGF-I axis have been demonstrated in CHF which may play a important role in the pathogenesis of the wasting process and therefore could have therapeutic implications [56]. There are elevated levels of growth hormone together with inappropriately normal or low levels of IGF-I in cachectic CHF patients, suggesting the presence of GH resistance [19]. Patients with low IGF-1 levels have evidence of abnormalities in body composition, cytokine and neuroendocrine activation, that are more severe than in patients with normal/high levels [57]. IGF-I inhibits apoptosis through receptor mediated inhibition of a number of intracellular caspases, the effector enzymes of the apoptosis pathway [58]. Apoptosis has been demonstrated in the skeletal muscle of patients with CHF, a finding which was shown to be associated with significant impairment of exercise capacity [59]. Although it is likely that apoptosis is particularly frequent in cardiac cachexia, this has not been studied as yet.

Clinical implications

The detection of wasting in a CHF patient is an ominous sign. As cardiac cachexia is a multifactorial disorder characterised by a complex imbalance of different body systems (Fig. 4), it is unlikely that any single agent will be completely effective in treating this condition and the targeting of different pathways will be necessary.

Nutritional support

It is clear that the nutritional status in cachectic patients has to be improved in order to regain energy reserves, thereby resulting in a gain in skeletal muscle tissue and a subsequent improvement of exercise capacity. To date, there have been no large controlled studies of nutritional strategies in cardiac cachexia. In stable CHF patients with no signs of severe malnutrition, nutritional support alone does not have a signifi-

cant effect on clinical status [60]. Although intensive nutritional support can increase the body's oxidative demands, it has been shown that this is safe in cachectic CHF patients and can lead to an increase in the amount of lean tissue [61]. This strategy is especially important in the pre- and postoperative state. Immediate postoperative intravenous hyperalimentation alone did not improve survival in one study [12], whereas in a separate study in which cachectic patients with heart failure received preoperative nutritional support (5–8 weeks duration, intravenously up to 1200 kcal/day) there was an improvement in the mortality rate in the treatment group (17% vs 57%, p < 0.05) [8]. The provision of 40–50 kcal/m^2 body surface/h including 1.5 to 2 g/kg/h protein, and sodium (2 g per day) and fluid (1000–1500 ml/day) restriction using high density continuous feeding has been proposed for CHF patients [12]. In the management of the cachectic CHF patient, specialist dietetic input is advisable.

Exercise

Muscular metabolic abnormalities and atrophy as well as impaired peripheral blood flow and neuro-

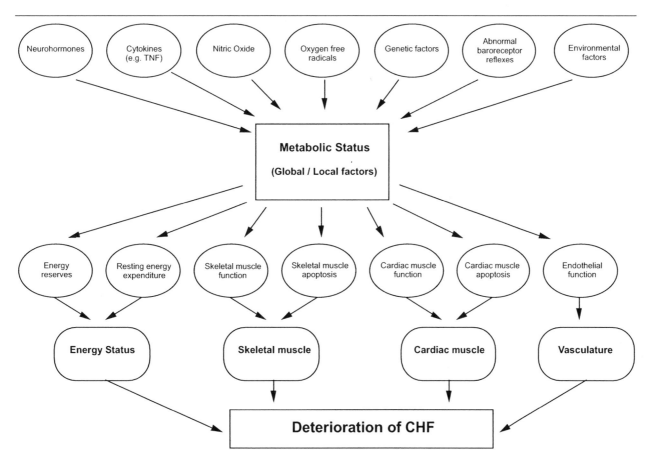

Fig. 4. *The complex interactions between different body systems in the pathogenesis of chronic heart failure. Adapted from [25].*

hormonal abnormalities can all be reversed by exercise rehabilitation training, leading to an improvement in exercise capacity [62]. We have previously shown that peak leg blood flow rather than muscle size and strength is the best correlate of impaired exercise capacity in cachectic CHF patients, whereas muscle strength and age are the best predictors of exercise intolerance in non-cachectic patients [49]. Whether this has implications for a potential systematic rehabilitation program (for instance the use of physiotherapeutic procedures to increase peripheral perfusion before the start of any exercise training) has not been studied to date.

Drug therapy

Previously, the drugs used to treat patients with CHF were aimed primarily at improving the hemodynamic indices in this condition. However, it is now clear that there is a poor correlation between hemodynamic parameters and patient symptoms and survival in CHF [63]. With increasing evidence that neurohormonal and immune pathways may play an important role in the pathophysioiogy of CHF, particularly cardiac cachexia, drugs which may beneficially modulate these systems are being developed.

Fish oil (n-3 polyunsaturated fatty acids) supplementation has been shown to reduce IL-1 concentrations and improve cachexia in dogs with congestive heart failure [64]. In this study a reduction in IL-1 levels predicted survival, suggesting that anticytokine therapies may be of benefit in patients with CHF. Specific anti-cytokine therapies have recently been introduced for the management of rheumatoid arthritis [65] and Crohns disease [66]. The value of such treatment in the management of CHF is currently being evaluated. In a pilot study, a soluble p75 TNF receptor fusion protein called etanercept (which essentially blocks the effects of TNF) was given to a small group of patients with NYHA class III heart failure and elevated TNF levels [67]. There were trends for increases in quality of life scores, 6-minute walk distance and ejection fraction, accompanied with a decrease in the biologically active levels of TNF. Recently, a randomized, double-blind, placebo-controlled trial of etanercept was performed in 47 patients with NYHA class III to IV heart failure [68]. Treatment with etarnercept for 3 months resulted in a significant improvement in left ventricular function and remodeling, together with a trend towards improvement in patient clinical status. Larger clinical trials are currently underway to assess the potential benefits of long-term etanercept therapy for CHF.

A recent study of immunoglobulin therapy in CHF demonstrated that a reduction of inflammatory cytokines (IL-1β) and an increase in anti-inflammatory mediators (IL-10 and IL-1 receptor antagonist) is possible [69]. However, no clinical benefit in terms of NYHA class or peak oxygen consumption were found, despite a trend for a small improvement in left ventricular ejection fraction (LVEF) in the actively treated group (LVEF $+5\%$, p $=0.08$ vs placebo).

Angiotensin II is a potent stimulator of both the immune and neurohormonal axes, and therefore it may be anticipated that treatment with ACE inhibitors and angiotensin II type I receptor antagonists would have important effects on these pathways that are thought to be important for the development of cachexia [19]. Furthermore, it has been shown that ACE inhibitors can restore depressed levels of circulating IGF-1 in patients with CHF, most likely by reducing angiotensin II activity [70]. Indeed, there is preliminary evidence that the ACE inhibitor enalarpil can prevent the development of weight loss in CHF patients [10]. Recently, Tsutamoto and colleagues investigated the effects of candesartan, an angiotensin II type I receptor antagonist, on immune markers in 23 patients with mild to moderate CHF. In this study it was demonstrated that candesartan therapy resulted in reduced plasma levels of TNF, IL-6, and BNP [71]. However, caution must be exercised when trying to interpret the significance of changes in the levels of immune and neurohormonal parameters. For example, although spironolactone (a competitive aldosterone receptor antagonist) is known to be beneficial in patients with CHF in terms of morbidity and mortality [72], this drug has been shown to augment neurohormonal activity [73].

On the anabolic side, recombinant human growth hormone may been considered an option for the treatment of cardiac cachexia, although normal doses (2 IU per day given daily) did not cause significant clinical benefits after 3 months of treatment compared to placebo [74]. Two case reports [75,76] demonstrated that short periods (1 week to 3 months) of high-dose GH therapy (70 to 98 IU per week) of 3 cachectic CHF patients resulted in profound increases of muscle mass and strength and improvement of exercise capacity with no reported side effects. The use of anabolic steroids to increase muscle mass may be an option, but their side effects (such as kidney function and the potential to induce prostate hyperplasia) may limit their potential unless substances are used with (nearly) no androgenic action.

Conclusions

Diseases that have a high priority in national health care programmes need to be i) common, ii) detectable, and iii) effectively treatable. Chronic heart failure has a prevalence of about 1–2% in the population which appears to be on the increase. Cachectic CHF patients represent a significant proportion of CHF patients, with this condition being readily detectable. A long-term aim is be to be able to predict the development of cardiac cachexia and to stop the wasting process before the onset of significant weight loss. Enhancing the prognosis of cardiac cachexia or even reversing the cachectic process will have a significant influence on the quality of life of many patients and may improve the long term prognosis of CHF overall.

Traditional ideas regarding the pathogenesis of CHF and the development of cardiac cachexia are proving to be inadequate as our understanding of the disease process improves. As a result, this has stimulated the search for other hypotheses to explain the systemic features of this condition. The immune and neurohormonal abnormalities present in CHF may play a significant role in the pathogenesis of the wasting process and it is hoped that further research into this area will lead to the development of new treatments for cardiac cachexia in the future. We regard this area of heart research as one of the most interesting as it requires a joint effort from cardiologists, endocrinologists and immunologists. Studying cardiac cachexia means studying metabolic cardiology.

References

1. Katz AM, Katz PB. Diseases of heart in works of Hippocrates. *Brit Heart J* 1962;24:257–264.
2. Anker SD, Coats AJS. Cardiac cachexia: a syndrome with impaired survival and immune and neuroendocrine activation. *Chest* 1999;115:836–847.
3. Metropolitan height and weight tables. Stat Bull Metrop Life Found 1983;64:3–9.
4. Anker SD, Ponikowski P, Varney S, Chua TP, Clark AL, Webb-Peploe KM, Harrington D, Kox WJ, Poole-Wilson PA, Coats AJ. Wasting as independent risk factor for mortality in chronic heart failure. *Lancet* 1997;349:1050–1053.
5. Carr JG, Stevenson LW, Walden JA, Heber D. Prevalence and haemodynamic correlates of malnutrition in severe congestive heart failure secondary to ischaemic or idiopathic dilated cardiomyopathy. *Am J Cardiol* 1989;63:709–713.
6. McMurray J, Abdullah I, Dargie HJ, Shapiro D. Increased concentrations of tumor necrosis factor in "cachectic" patients with severe chronic heart failure. *Br Heart J* 1991;66:356–358.
7. Levine B, Kalman J, Mayer L, Fillit H, Packer M. Elevated circulating levels of tumor necrosis factor in severe chronic heart failure. *N Engl J Med* 1990;323:236–241.
8. Otaki M. Surgical treatment of patients with cardiac cachexia. An analysis of factors affecting operative mortality. *Chest* 1994;105:1347–1351.
9. Freeman LM, Roubenoff R. The nutrition implications of cardiac cachexia. *Nutr Rev* 1994;52:340–347.
10. Anker S, Negassa A, Coats A, Poole-Wilson P, Yusuf S. Weight loss in chronic heart failure (CHF) and the impact of treatment with ACE inhibitors – Results from the SOLVD treatment trial. *Circulation* 1999;100:I-781 (abstract).
11. Cowie MR, Mosterd A, Wood DA, Deckers JW, Poole-Wilson PA, Sutton GC, Grobbee DE. The epidemiology of heart failure. *Eur Heart J* 1997;18:208–225.
12. Abel RM, Fischer J, Buckley MJ, Barnett GO, Austen WG. Malnutrition in cardiac surgical patients. *Arch Surg* 1976;111:45–50.
13. Ansari A. Syndromes of cardiac cachexia and the cachectic heart: current perspective. *Progress in cardiovascular diseases* 1987;XXX:45–60.
14. Pittman JG, Cohen P. The pathogenesis of cardiac cachexia. *N Engl J Med* 1964;271:403–409.
15. Buchanan N, Keen RD, Kingsley R, Eyberg CD. Gastrointestinal absorption studies in cardiac cachexia. *Intensive Care Med* 1977;3:89–91.
16. King D, Smith ML, Chapman TJ, Stockdale HR, Lye M. Fat malabsorption in elderly patients with cardiac cachexia. *Age Ageing* 1996;25:144–149.
17. Braunwald E. Clinical manifestation of heart failure. In: *Heart disease. A textbook of cardiovascular medicine.* Vol. 1. Philadelphia, Saunders 1984:499.
18. MacGowan G, Mann D, Kormos R, Feldman A, Murali S. Circulating interleukin-6 in severe heart failure. *Am J Cardiol* 1997;79:1128–1131.
19. Anker SD, Chua TP, Ponikowski P, Harrington D, Swan JW, Kox WJ, Poole-Wilson PA, Coats AJ. Hormonal changes and catabolic/anabolic imbalance in chronic heart failure and their importance for cardiac cachexia. *Circulation* 1997;96:526–534.
20. Mancini DM, Walter G, Reichek N, Lenkinski R, McCuliy KK, Mullen JL, et al. Contribution of skeletal muscle atrophy to exercise intolerance and altered muscle metabolism in heart failure. *Circulation* 1992;85:1364–1373.
21. Vescovo G, Serafini F, Facchin L, Tenderini P, Carraro U, Della Libera L, et al. Specific changes in skeletal muscle myosin heavy chains composition in cardiac failure: differences compared with disuse atrophy as assessed on microbiopsies by high resolution electrophoresis. *Heart* 1996;76:337–343.
22. Poehlman ET, Scheffers J, Gottlieb SS, Fisher ML, Vaitekevicius P. Increased resting metabolic rate in patients with congestive heart failure. *Ann Intern Med* 1994;121:860–862.
23. Toth MJ, Gottlieb SS, Goran MI, Fisher ML, Poehlman ET. Daily energy expenditure in free-living heart failure patients. *Am J Physiol* 1997;272:E469–475.
24. Poehlman ET, Danforth E. Endurance training increases metabolic rate and norepinephrine appearance rate in older individuals. *Am J Physiol* 1991;261:E233–239.

25. Sharma R, Coats AJ, Anker SD. The role of inflammatory mediators in chronic heart failure: cytokines, nitric oxide, and endothelin-1. *Int J Cardiol* 2000;72:175–186.

26. Dutka DP, Elborn JS, Delamere F, Shale DJ, Morris GK. Tumour necrosis factor alpha in severe congestive cardiac failure. *Br Heart J* 1993;70:141–143.

27. Torre-Amione G, Kapadia S, Lee J, Durand JB, Bies RD, Young JB, Mann DL. Tumor necrosis factor-alpha and tumor necrosis factor receptors in the failing human heart. *Circulation* 1996;93:704–711.

28. Anker SD, Egerer KR, Volk HD, Kox WJ, Poole-Wilson PA, Coats AJ. Elevated soluble CD 14 receptors and altered cytokines in chronic heart failure. *Am J Cardiol* 1997;79:1426–1430.

29. Niebauer J, Volk HD, Kemp M, Dominguez M, Schumann RR, Rauchhaus M, Poole-Wilson PA, Coats AJS, Anker SD. Endotoxin and immune activation in chronic heart failure: a prospective cohort study. *Lancet* 1999;353:1838–1842.

30. Hasper D, Hummel M, Kleber FX, Reindl I, Volk HD. Systemic inflammation in patients with heart failure. *Eur Heart J* 1998;19:761–765.

31. Tracey KJ, Morgello S, Koplin B, Fahey TJ, Fox K, Aledo A. Metabolic effects of cachectin/tumor necrosis factor are modified by site of production: Cachectin/tumor necrosis factor-secreting tumor in skeletal muscle induces chronic cachexia, while implantation in brain induces predominantely acute cachexia. *J Clin Invest* 1990;86:2014–2024.

32. Anker SD, Voiterrani M, Egerer KR, Feiton CV, Kox WJ, Poole-Wilson PA, Coats AJ. Tumour necrosis factor alpha as a predictor of impaired peak leg blood flow in patients with chronic heart failure. *QJM* 1998;91:199–203.

33. Zumbach MS, Boehme MW, Wahl P, Stremmei W, Ziegler R, Nawroth PP. Tumor necrosis factor increases serum leptin levels in humans. *J Clin Endocrinol Metab* 1997;82:4080–4082.

34. Leyva F, Anker SD, Egerer K, Stevenson JC, Kox WJ, Coats AJ. Hyperleptinaemia in chronic heart failure. Relationships with insulin. *Eur Heart J* 1998;19:1547–1551.

35. Murdoch DR, Rooney E, Dargie HJ, Shapiro D, Morton JJ, McMurray JJ. Inappropriately low plasma leptin concentration in the cachexia associated with chronic heart failure. *Heart* 1999;82:352–356.

36. Torre-Amione G, Kapadia S, Benedict C, Oral H, Young JB, Mann DL. Proinflammatory cytokine levels in patients with depressed left ventricular ejection fraction: a report from the Studies of Left Ventricular Dysfunction (SOLVD). *J Am Coll Cardiol* 1996;27:1201–1206.

37. Rauchhaus M, Doehner W, Francis DP, Davos C, Kemp M, Liebenthal C, Niebauer J, Hooper J, Volk HD, Coats AJ, Anker SD. Plasma cytokine parameters and mortality in patients with chronic heart failure. *Circulation* 2000;102:3060–3067.

38. Sharma R, Rauchhaus M, Ponikowski PP, Varney S, Poole-Wilson PA, Mann DL, Coats AJ, Anker SD. The relationship of the erythrocyte sedimentation rate to inflammatory cytokines and survival in patients with chronic heart failure treated with angiotensin-converting enzyme inhibitors. *J Am Coll Cardiol* 2000;36:523–528.

39. Leyva F, Anker SD, Godsland IF, Teixeira M, Hellewell PG, Kox WJ, Poole-Wilson PA, Coats AJ. Uric acid in chronic heart failure: a marker of chronic inflammation. *Eur Heart J* 1998;19:1814–1822.

40. Packer M. The neurohormonal hypothesis: a theory to explain the mechanism of disease progression in heart failure. *J Am Coll Cardiol* 1992;20:248–254.

41. Chidsey CA, Harrison DC, Braunwald E. The augmentation of plasma norepinephrine response to exercise in patients with congestive heart failure. *New Engl J Med* 1962;267:650–654.

42. Brink M, Wellen J, Delafontaine P. Angiotensin II causes weight loss and decreases circulating insulin-like growth factor I in rats through a pressor-independent mechanism. *J Clin Invest* 1996;97:2509–2516.

43. Ponikowski P, Piepoli M, Chua TP, Banasiak W, Francis D, Anker SD, Coats AJ. The impact of cachexia on cardiorespiratory reflex control in chronic heart failure. *Eur Heart J* 1999;20:1667–1675.

44. Obisesan TO, Toth MJ, Donaldson K, Gottlieb SS, Fisher ML, Vaitekevicius P, Poehlman ET. Energy expenditure and symptom severity in men with heart failure. *Am J Cardiol* 1996;77:1250–1252.

45. Anker SD, Clark AL, Kemp M, Salsbury C, Teixeira MM, Hellewell PG, Coats AJ. Tumor necrosis factor and steroid metabolism in chronic heart failure: possible relation to muscle wasting. *J Am Coll Cardiol* 1997;30:997–1001.

46. Lipkin DP, Jones DA, Round JM, Poole-Wilson PA. Abnormalities of skeletal muscle in patients with chronic heart failure. *Int J Cardiol* 1988;18:187–195.

47. Drexler H, Riede U, Munzel T, Konig H, Funke E, Just H. Alterations of skeletal muscle in chronic heart failure. *Circulation* 1992;85:1751–1759.

48. Harrington D, Anker SD, Chua TP, Webb-Peploe KM, Ponikowski PP, Poole-Wilson PA, Coats AJ. Skeletal muscle function and its relation to exercise tolerance in chronic heart failure. *J Am Coll Cardiol* 1997;30:1758–1764.

49. Anker SD, Swan JW, Volterrani M, Chua TP, Clark AL, Poole-Wilson PA, Coats AJ. The influence of muscle mass, strength, fatigability and blood flow on exercise capacity in cachectic and non-cachectic patients with chronic heart failure. *Eur Heart J* 1997;18:259–269.

50. Kotler DP, Tierney AR, Wang J, Pierson RN. Magnitude of body-cell-mass depletion and the timing of death from wasting in AIDS. *Am J Clin Nutr* 1989;50:444–447.

51. Thomas RD, Silverton NP, Burkinshaw L, Morgan DB. Potassium depletion and tissue loss in chronic heart disease. *Lancet* 1979;310:9–11.

52. Anker SD, Harrington D, Lees B, Chua TP, Ponikowski P, Poole-Wilson PA, Coats A. Body composition and quality of muscle in chronic heart failure. *J Am Coll Cardiol* 1997;29:527A (Abstract).

53. Anker SD, Clark AL, Teixeira MM, Hellewell PG, Coats AJ. Loss of bone mineral in patients with cachexia due to chronic heart failure. *Am J Cardiol* 1999;83:612–615, Al0.

54. Volterrani M, Clark AL, Ludman PF, Swan JW, Adamopoulos S, Piepoli M, Coats AJ. Predictors of exercise capacity in chronic heart failure. *Eur Heart J* 1994;15:801–809.

55. Anker SD, Ponikowski PP, Clark AL, Leyva F, Rauchhaus M, Kemp M, Teixeira MM, Hellewell PG,

Hooper J, PooleWilson PA, Coats AJ. Cytokines and neurohormones relating to body composition alterations in the wasting syndrome of chronic heart failure. *Eur Heart J* 1999;20:683–693.

56. Volterrani M, Manelli F, Cicoira M, Lorusso R, Giustina A. Role of growth hormone in chronic heart failure. Therapeutic implications. *Drugs* 2000;60: 711–719.

57. Niebauer J, Pflaum CD, Clark AL, Strasburger CJ, Hooper J, Poole-Wilson PA, Coats AJ, Anker SD. Deficient insulin-like growth factor I in chronic heart failure predicts altered body composition, anabolic deficiency, cytokine and neurohormonal activation. *J Am Coll Cardiol* 1998;32:393–397.

58. Werner H, Stannard B, Bach MA, Roberts CT Jr, LeRoith D. Regulation of insulin-like growth factor I receptor gene expression in normal and pathological states. *Adv Exp Med Biol* 1991;293:263–272.

59. Adams V, Jiang H, Jiangtao Y, Mobius-Winider S, Fiehn E, Linke A, Weigl C, Schuler G, Hambrecht R. Apoptosis in skeletal myocytes of patients with chronic heart failure is associated with exercise intolerance. *J Am Coll Cardiol* 1999;33:959–965.

60. Broquist M, Arnquist H, Dahlström U, Larsson J, Nylander E, Permert J. Nutritional assessment and muscle energy metabolism in severe chronic congestive heart failure-effects of long-term dietary supplementation. *Europ Heart J* 1994;15:1641–1650.

61. Heymsfield SB, Casper K. Congestive heart failure: clinical management by use of continuous nasoenteric feeding. *Am J Clin Nutr* 1989;50:539–544.

62. Coats AJ, Adamopoulos S, Meyer TE, Conway J, Sleight P. Effects of physical training in chronic heart failure. *Lancet* 1990;335:63–66.

63. Clark AL, Poole-Wilson PA, Coats AJ. Exercise limitation in chronic heart failure: central role of the periphery. *J Am Coll Cardiol* 1996;28:1092–1102.

64. Freeman L, Rush J, Kehayias J, Ross J Jr, Meydani S, Brown D, Dolnikowski G, Marmor B, White M, Dinarello C, Roubenoff R. Nutritional alterations and the effect of fish oil supplementation in dogs with heart failure. *J Vet Intern Med* 1998;12:440–448.

65. Moreland LW. Inhibitors of tumor necrosis factor for rheumatoid arthritis. *J Rheumatol* 1999;26:7–15.

66. Present DH, Rutgeerts P, Targan S, Hanauer SB, Mayer L, van Hogezand RA, Podolsky DK, Sands BE, Braakman T, DeWoody KL, Schaible TF, van Deventer SJ. Infliximab for the treatment of fistulas in patients with Crohn's disease. *N Engl J Med* 1999;340:1398–1405.

67. Deswal A, Bozkurt B, Seta Y, Parilti-Eiswirth S, Hayes F, Blosch C, Mann D. Safety and efficacy of a soluble P75 tumor necrosis factor receptor (Enbrel, etanercept) in patients with advanced heart failure. *Circulation* 1999;99:3224–3226.

68. Bozkurt B, Torre-Amione G, Warren MS, Whitmore J, Soran OZ, Feldman AM, Mann DL. Results of targeted anti-tumor necrosis factor therapy with etanercept (ENBREL) in patients with advanced heart failure. *Circulation* 2001;103:1044–1047.

69. Gullestad L, Aass H, Fjeld JG, Wikeby L, Andreassen AK, Ihlen H, Simonsen S, Kjekshus J, Nitter-Hauge S, Ueland T, Lien E, Froland SS, Aukrust P. Immunomodulating therapy with intravenous immunoglobulin in patients with chronic heart failure. *Circulation* 2001;103:220–225.

70. Corbalan R, Acevedo M, Godoy I, Jalil J, Campusano C, Klassen J. Enalapril restores depressed circulating insulin-like growth factor 1 in patients with chronic heart failure. *J Card Fail* 1998;4:115–119.

71. Tsutamoto T, Wada A, Maeda K, Mabuchi N, Hayashi M, Tsutsui T, Ohnishi M, Sawaki M, Fujii M, Matsumoto T, Kinoshita M. Angiotensin II type 1 receptor antagonist decreases plasma levels of tumor necrosis factor alpha, interleukin-6 and soluble adhesion molecules in patients with chronic heart failure. *J Am Coll Cardiol* 2000;35:714–721.

72. Pitt B, Zannad F, Renime WJ, Cody R, Castaigne A, Perez A, Palensky J, Wittes J. The effect of spironolactone on morbidity and mortality in patients with severe heart failure. Randomized Aldactone Evaluation Study Investigators. *N Engl J Med* 1999;34 1:709–717.

73. Kinugawa T, Ogino K, Kato M, Furuse Y, Shimoyama M, Mon M, Endo A, Kato T, Omodani H, Osaki S, Miyakoda H, Hisatome I, Shigemasa C. Effects of spironolactone on exercise capacity and neurohormonal factors in patients with heart failure treated with loop diuretics and angiotensin-converting enzyme inhibitor. *Gen Pharmacol* 1998;31:93–99.

74. Osterziel KJ, Strohm O, Schuler J, Friedrich M, Hanlein D, Willenbrock R, Anker SD, Poole-Wilson PA, Ranke MB, Dietz R. Randomised, double-blind, placebo-controlled trial of human recombinant growth hormone in patients with chronic heart failure due to dilated cardiomyopathy. *Lancet* 1998; 351:1233–1237.

75. Cuneo RC, Wilmshurst P, Lowy C, McGauley G, Sonksen PH. Cardiac failure responding to growth hormone. *Lancet* 1989;1:838–839.

76. O'Driscoll JG, Green DJ, Ireland M, Kerr D, Larbalestier RI. Treatment of end-stage cardiac failure with growth hormone. *Lancet* 1997;349:1068.

INDEX